Quick Reference Glossary of Eye Care Terminology
Second Edition

Quick Reference Glossary of Eyecare Terminology
Second Edition

Joseph Hoffman
Editor in Chief
Ocular Surgery News
Ocular Surgery News International Edition
Primary Care Optometry News

The Basic Bookshelf for Eyecare
Professionals
Series Editors: Janice K. Ledford, Ken
Daniels, Robert Campbell

SLACK Incorporated, 6900 Grove Road,
Thorofare, NJ 08086

Publisher: John H. Bond
Editorial Director: Amy E. Drummond
Senior Associate Editor: Jennifer J. Cahill
Creative Director: Linda Baker

ISBN 1-55642-370-5

Printed in the United States of America
Published by: SLACK Incorporated
                       6900 Grove Road
                       Thorofare, NJ 08086-9447 USA
                       Telephone: 609-848-1000
                       Fax: 609-853-5991
                       World Wide Web: http://www.slackinc.com

Last digit is print number: 10 9 8 7 6 5 4 3 2 1

Dedication

To Joe Sr. and Etta Hoffman, because Dad asked
me why I didn't in the first book.

Contents

How to Use This Glossary

Abbreviations: Spelled out so they can be found in the glossary. Abbreviations are not duplicated in the main text of the glossary, but all of the spelled-out forms of these abbreviations (except company and trade names, professional society names and certification credentials) are defined. Look up abbreviations on pages 215 through 224 to find corresponding entry word and definition in text.

Text: Defining the ophthalmic terms most often used in eyecare clinics and literature. Compound words are alphabetized as if they were single, unpunctuated words (achromatopsia comes before A-constant). Compound words are usually defined under the form most commonly used in eyecare, but reader should look under main noun if the compound is not found. Some compound words have only a cross-reference to the main noun when several related compound words must be defined. For example, cystoid macular edema is a main entry (not edema), but age-related macular degeneration, dry macular degeneration, etc., are all cross-referenced as "see macular degeneration." Except for these cross-referenced compound words, words with full definitions are more commonly used than those that have only a cross-reference. Related terms are referenced in

definitions by "see also," antonyms by "compare."
The style in this book is for eponyms identifying
anatomic structures to be given with 's, while
those identifying diseases, syndromes,
phenomena, tests, etc., are given without 's. The
most common combining forms (typically Latin
and Greek roots) that are specifically ophthalmic
are included. With very few exceptions, trade
names are not included, as they tend to be
ephemeral. Other words not found in this glossary
(especially the many Latin synonyms for the
English terms given here) will probably be found
in a general dictionary or medical reference book
such as *Dorland's Illustrated Medical Dictionary*
(published by WB Saunders Co).

Aa

abducens nerve sixth cranial nerve, innervating the lateral rectus muscle

abduct general medical term for inducing motion away from the center of the body; in ophthalmic usage, muscles that move an eye toward the temple are called abductors; compare **adduct**

aberration uneven refraction of light in an optical system resulting in distortion of the transmitted image; see also **chromatic aberration** and **spherical aberration**

ab externo general medical term meaning *from the outside*; in ophthalmic usage, describing surgical procedures in which the approach to an anatomic structure is made from outside the globe

ablation general medical term for destruction (usually as part of a surgical procedure) of tissue; in laser surgery, vaporization of tissue by the laser

ablatio retinae see **retinal detachment**

ablepharia, -on, -y congenital absence or diminishment in size of eyelids

ablepsia, -y see **blindness**

abnormal retinal correspondence see **anomalous retinal correspondence**

abrasion general medical term for wound in which layers of tissue are scraped away; in ophthalmic usage, often used as a synonym for **corneal abrasion**

accommodation adjustment of focal power of the eye from distance to near vision, achieved by contraction of the ciliary muscle, which causes a thickening of the crystalline lens and a slight forward shift in its position, both of which increase its refractive power; **absolute a.** accommodation of either eye independently; **binocular a.** uniform accommodation of both eyes together in convergence (the inward turning of both eyes in viewing a near object); **convergence a.** accommodation that occurs in either eye upon convergence; **far point of a.** distance from the eye to the farthest point clearly visible when accommodation is relaxed; **near point of a.** distance from the eye to the nearest point clearly visible when accommodation is at its maximum; **negative a.** relaxation of accommodation for distance vision; **positive a.** exercise of accommodation for near vision; **range of a.** the distance between the near and far points of accommodation

accommodation amplitude total range of accommodation (measured in diopters) from distance to near vision to which the eye can adjust

accommodative convergence inward turning of both eyes that normally occurs in response to accommodation

accommodative convergence/accommodation ratio relationship between the amount that the eyes turn inward (accommodative convergence, measured in prism diopters) and the increase in their focusing power (accommodation, measured in diopters) occurring upon viewing a near object, calculated as accommodative convergence divided by accommodation; abbreviation: AC/A ratio

accommodative insufficiency weakening of the accommodation reflex due to injury, disease or the effects of medication

accommodative miosis normal constriction of pupils associated with accommodation

accommodative spasm accommodation without subsequent relaxation of the ciliary muscle, resulting in a prolonged state of near focus, pupil constriction and convergence

achromatic lens lens that is free from chromatic aberration; that is, it does not break light into its component colors

achromatopia, -sia see **monochromatism**

A-constant 1. number assigned to an intraocular lens (IOL) by the manufacturer based on the lens design, used in formulas for calculating power of IOL needed in a given patient; 2. number derived from actual visual results of IOL implantation by a particular surgeon, used as part of subsequent IOL power calculations to "personalize" formula and better reflect the influence of surgeon technique

acorea absence of the pupil

acrylic of or relating to acrylic acid or its many derivative compounds; in eyecare, usually an optically clear polymer used in manufacture of lenses

acrylic lens implant see **intraocular lens**

acuity clarity of vision; specifically, the ability to distinguish fine details; often expressed as a score on Snellen, Jaeger, or other vision testing charts

acute in medical usage, denoting the immediate or severe (compare **chronic**); see entries under main word, as in **acute angle-closure glaucoma** see **glaucoma,** etc.

adaptation general medical term for adjustment to changing conditions; specifically in ophthalmic usage: **color a.** adjustment of vision to bright colors such that the color intensity diminishes with time; **dark a.** adjustment of vision in dim light, primarily by increasing levels of rhodopsin (visual purple) in the rods of the retina, making the eye more sensitive to light (see **scotopia**); **light a.** adjustment of vision in bright light by decreasing levels of light-sensitive pigments of the retina (see **photopia**); **photopic a.** see **light a.; retinal a.** general term for adjustment of vision to varying light conditions; **scotopic a.** see **dark a.**

add 1. amount of additional refractive power needed in spectacles or contact lenses prescribed for distance vision correction to correct a presbyopic eye to near ("reading") vision; 2. the portion of a lens that is designed to provide that additional near corrective power; see also **segment**

adduct general medical term for inducing motion toward the center of the body; in ophthalmic usage, muscles that move an eye toward the nose are called adductors; compare **abduct**

Adie pupil or **syndrome** uneven contraction of the pupils of each eye upon accommodation in near vision

adjustable suture suture placed in glaucoma, refractive or other surgery to allow tightening or loosening in postoperative period to modify the results of surgery

adnexa general anatomic term for the structures surrounding an organ; the ocular adnexa are usually considered to include the eyelids, lacrimal apparatus, orbits and other tissues within the orbits

advancement in ophthalmic usage, operation (usually for correction of strabismus) in which an extraocular muscle or tendon is detached and repositioned more anteriorly to increase its action; **capsular a.** surgical manipulation of Tenon's capsule in order to achieve advancement of an extraocular muscle

afferent defect in ophthalmic usage, impairment of nerve function that results in Marcus Gunn pupil

after-cataract see **cataract**

afterimage perception of an image that persists after the visual stimulus ends; **complementary a.** afterimage in which the persisting colors are complementary to the colors of the original visual stimulus; **negative a.** afterimage in which bright elements of a visual stimulus persist as dark and dark elements become light; **positive a.** afterimage in which light elements persist as light and dark elements remain dark

against-the-rule astigmatism see **astigmatism**

age-related macular degeneration see **macular degeneration**

agnosia inability to recognize familiar objects on sight

agraphia inability to express ideas in writing

air-fluid exchange see **gas-fluid exchange**

air-puff tonometer see **tonometer**

akinesia general term for lack of motion or inability to move; most often in ophthalmic usage, referring to impossibility of voluntary movement of the eye following retrobulbar or peribulbar anesthesia

alexia inability to understand written language

Allen cards, chart or **test** visual acuity test employing pictures to assess the vision of young children

allergic conjunctivitis see **conjunctivitis**

alpha angle see **angle**

alpha chymotrypsin enzyme injected into the anterior chamber to dissolve zonular fibers and facilitate intracapsular cataract extraction

alternate cover test see **cover test**

alternating amblyopia and **strabismus** see entries under each main word

amacrine cells nerve cells found in the inner nuclear layer of the retina

amaurosis general term for blindness, usually referring to blindness caused by some defect apart from the tissues of the eyeball; **central a.** temporary blindness resulting from disease or defect of the central nervous system; **hysterical a.** temporary blindness resulting from neurosis; **sympathetic a.** blindness in one eye occurring because of disease in the other eye

amaurosis fugax a temporary (about ten minutes or so) state of partial or full blindness in one eye

amaurotic nystagmus rapid involuntary movements of a blind eye

amaurotic pupil pupil that does not respond to direct light stimulation but does dilate and constrict when the fellow eye receives light stimulus; an eye with an amaurotic pupil is blind, usually because of damage to the optic nerve or retina

amblyope one who suffers from amblyopia

amblyopia impaired vision in one or both eyes that cannot be remedied with corrective lenses and has no obvious organic cause in the structures of the eye or visual pathway (colloquially known as "lazy eye"); **alcoholic a.** amblyopia caused by alcohol toxicity (also known as *amblyopia crapulosa*); **alternating a.** diminished vision occurring in the non-fixating eye in alternating strabismus; **ametropic a.** see **refractive a.; anisometropic a.** amblyopia arising from a difference in the refractive power of the two eyes in which the eye requiring the greatest accommodation to achieve clear vision becomes disused; **astigmatic a.** refractive amblyopia occurring because of uncorrected astigmatism; **color a.** general term for impairment of color vision; **crossed a.** amblyopia in one eye with loss of feeling in the opposite side of the face (also known as *amblyopia cruciata*); **deprivation a.** amblyopia following a period in which central fixation was lost due to cataract, drooping eyelid, etc. (also known as *amblyopia of disuse*), called **occlusion a.** when central fixation was intentionally obstructed (as with an eye patch); **functional** or **reversible a.** amblyopia that can be corrected by eyeglasses or occlusion of the opposite eye in childhood; **nocturnal a.** see **nyctalopia; reflex a.** amblyopia resulting from some insult or injury to the eye; **refractive a.** amblyopia in an eye that has a large uncorrected refractive error or amblyopia caused by a difference in the refraction between the two eyes (more correctly called **anisometropic a.**); **strabismic a.** amblyopia arising from strabismus in which one eye becomes preferred over the other, which then falls into disuse; **suppression a.** amblyopia resulting from deprivation of sight in an eye by ptosis, cataract, corneal opacity, etc.; also called *amblyopia ex anopsia* or *amblyopia of disuse*

ametropia general term for conditions in which the eye does not focus properly but can be corrected with eyeglasses or other vision aids (see **astigmatism, hyperopia, myopia** and **presbyopia**); **axial a.** ametropia attributable to the length of the eyeball (too long in myopia or too short in hyperopia); **curvature a.** ametropia attributable to corneal curvature (too steep in myopia or too flat in hyperopia); **position a.** ametropia attributable to the position of the crystalline lens of the eye (too far forward in myopia or too far back in hyperopia); **refractive a.** general term for any ametropia attributable to error in the eye's system for focusing light rays on the retina; compare **emmetropia**

amplitude of accommodation see **accommodation**

amplitude of convergence maximum angle to which the eyes can turn inward (from parallel lines of sight in distance vision) toward the nose to fix upon a nearby object

Amsler grid vision test target consisting of evenly spaced horizontal and vertical lines, typically white lines on a dark background with a central dot to mark the point of fixation; used as a simple test for detecting defects or distortions of the central visual field

amyloid body deposit of abnormal starch-protein compound seen in amyloidosis

amyloidosis condition in which deposits of amyloid accumulate in various body tissues, including the vitreous humor and ocular nerves and blood vessels

anaclasimeter instrument for measuring the refractive power of the eye

anaclasis general term for the reflection or refraction of light rays

anaglyph vision test target consisting of two similar images with different portions printed in red, green and sometimes black; subject views each image separately with each eye, and a red filter is placed before one eye and a green filter before the other; patient reports the image seen, providing a measure of fusion and stereoscopic function

anatomic equator in ophthalmic usage, imaginary line around the circumference of the eyeball placed equidistant from the front and back surfaces (anterior and posterior poles) of the eyeball

angioid streaks red to brown streaks originating from the optic disk on fundoscopic examination

angioscotoma visual field defect caused by the shadow of a retinal blood vessel

angle 1. the point at which the upper and lower eyelids meet (see also **canthus**); 2. the area of the anterior chamber of the eye where the iris and cornea join (also called the **iridocorneal angle**); aqueous humor exits the eye through the angle, thus this structure is also called the

filtration angle; specific tissues and structures that comprise the angle include the iris processes, corneoscleral junction, scleral sulcus, ciliary body, trabecular meshwork and Schlemm's canal; 2. any one of several standard measurements used to describe the optical system of the eye, specifically: **alpha a.** angle formed at the eye's optical center by the optical and visual axes; **biorbital a.** angle formed by the axes of the two orbits; **gamma a.** angle formed at the eye's center of rotation by the optical and fixation axes; **kappa a.** angle formed at the eye's optical center by the pupillary and visual axes; **lambda a.** angle formed at the center of the eye's pupil by the optical and the visual axes; see also **axis** and **optical center**

angle-closure glaucoma see **glaucoma**

angle of anomaly discrepancy between patient's report of normal vision and the objective measurement of deviation in the alignment of the eyes

angle of convergence angle formed by the eye's visual axis and a line drawn from the target object to a midpoint between the two eyes

angle of deviation degree to which one eye is shifted from straight-ahead fixation when the fellow eye is fixed straight ahead

angle of direction degree to which the eye must be turned to bring an image onto the fovea

angle of incidence angle formed by a ray of light that strikes (is "incident" to) an interface between two media, as measured from a line drawn perpendicular to the interface at the point where the light ray strikes

angle of reflection angle formed by a ray of light reflected from the interface of two media, as measured from a line drawn perpendicular to the interface at the point from which the light ray is reflected

angle of refraction angle formed by a ray of light that has crossed an interface between two substances and a line drawn perpendicular to the interface at the point where the light ray crosses

angle-recession glaucoma see **glaucoma**

aniridia absence (sometimes congenital, though more frequently due to trauma in adults) of most or all of the iris

aniseikonia condition in which the image from an object is focused larger on one retina than on the other, resulting in distortions of perceived spatial relations

anisoaccommodation general term for uneven accommodation in the two eyes

anisochromatic color difference, either between two or more objects (as in some vision test targets for color blindness) or between different parts of the same object (as in an iris that is not of a uniform color); see also **heterochromic**

anisocoria uneven size of pupils in the two eyes, usually reserved to describe more than a 1-mm difference in diameter

anisometropia uneven refractive power of the two eyes, usually connoting more than a 1-diopter difference

anisophoria heterophoria in which there is uneven deviation between the two eyes depending on which eye is occluded

anisopia general term for unequal vision in the two eyes

ankyloblepharon adhesion of the upper and lower eyelids

annular ring-shaped

annular cataract see **cataract**

annular keratitis see **keratitis**

annular scotoma see **scotoma**

annulus general anatomic term for a ring-shaped structure

annulus ciliaris outer portion of the ciliary body attached to the ora serrata

annulus of Zinn ring of connective tissue attached to the orbit near the optic nerve, anchoring the rectus muscles of the eye (also called the **aponeurosis**)

anomalous retinal correspondence condition in which parts of the images on each retina come to be linked in the brain's interpretation of the fused image, even though they do not correspond to the same point in space, often occurring a result of untreated strabismus; compare **harmonious retinal correspondence**

anomalous trichromatism condition in which there is a deficiency of some of the three types of photosensitive pigments found in the cones of the retina

anophthalmia, -os, anopia congenital condition in which the eyeball is absent or only partially developed

anopsia loss or suppression of vision, usually of only part of the visual field in just one eye

anorthopia general term for distortion of vision

anotropia condition in which the eyes shift so that the gaze is fixed above the target object

anterior basal membrane see **Bowman's membrane**

anterior chamber area within the eye formed by the structures forward of the iris and lens-zonule apparatus that contains the aqueous humor; compare **posterior chamber**

anterior hyaloid membrane see **hyaloid membrane**

anterior pole of the eye imaginary point on the front surface of the cornea centered over the pupil; compare **posterior pole of the eye**

anterior pole of the lens point at the front and center of the crystalline lens; compare **posterior pole of the lens**

anterior segment of the eye general term usually describing the structures of the eye lying in front of the plane of the iris but also including the lens-zonule apparatus and ciliary body; ophthalmic surgery is roughly divided into the categories of anterior segment (cornea, glaucoma and cataract procedures) and posterior segment (retina and vitreous procedures)

anterior synechiae adhesions (singular: synechia) of the iris to the cornea; may be referred to as peripheral anterior synechiae

anterior uveitis inflammation of the iris and ciliary body

anterior vitrectomy see **vitrectomy**

antimetropia condition in which one eye is hyperopic while the fellow eye is myopic; also called heterometropia

antimydriatic drug that prevents the pupil from dilating

A pattern esotropia see **esotropia**

aphake one in whom the lens of the eye is absent, either congenitally or following surgery

aphakia absence of the lens of the eye; see cataract extraction

aphakic contact lenses or spectacles vision correction devices prescribed after removal of the crystalline lens of the eye; see also **cataract extraction**

aphakic glaucoma elevated intraocular pressure after removal of the crystalline lens of the eye; see also **cataract extraction**

aphotesthesia diminished response of the retina following excessive exposure to bright light

apical clearance 1. distance between the back surface of a contact lens and the cornea; 2. less commonly, distance between the cornea and the crystalline lens

aplanatic, -ism property of an optical system such that it is free of the aberrations normally associated with spherical lenses

aponeurosis general term for the tendon that anchors a muscle; in the eye, the tendinous bundle that anchors the rectus muscles to the orbit (also called the **annulus of Zinn**)

apoptosis general medical term for "programmed cell death," a process by which cells continue to degenerate and cease functioning long after the initial injury or insult; in ophthalmic usage, usually referring to the progressive loss of retinal cells in glaucoma

apotripsis surgical excision of corneal opacity

applanation flattening of a normally rounded area, such as the cornea

applanation tonometer see **tonometer**

applanometer see **applanation tonometer** under **tonometer**

aqueous flare see **flare**

aqueous fluid or **humor** clear, watery liquid (typically referred to simply as the aqueous) that fills the anterior chamber of the eye

aqueous outflow process by which the aqueous humor is filtered out of the eye through the ciliary body; see also definition 2 under **angle**

arachnoid sheath one of the membranes that surround the optic nerve

arcuate scotoma see **scotoma**

arcus juvenilis ring of fatty deposits around the edge of the cornea but not quite extending to the limbus, appearing in young or middle-aged patients with unusually high blood cholesterol levels or some systemic diseases

arcus senilis ring of fatty deposits around the edge of the cornea but not quite extending to the limbus, appearing in elderly patients

argon laser see **laser**

Argyll Robertson pupil condition in which a pupil constricts upon accommodation but does not react to varying light levels

arterial circles of the iris two ring-shaped bands of vascular tissue in the iris: the inner or lesser circle is near the pupil and the major or greater circle is adjacent to the ciliary body

arthro-ophthalmopathy degenerative disease that affects the joints and eyes

artificial tears man-made liquid formulated to simulate the composition of tear fluid, used in treating dry eye conditions

A-scan as used in ophthalmology, an ultrasound examination to determine the axial length of the eye (distance from front of cornea to back of retina) and possibly the depth of various intraocular structures; most commonly used in calculating the power of intraocular lenses

aspheric, -al curved surface, typically in ophthalmic usage the surface of a lens, whose cross section in some directions is non-circular; aspheric optics are used in spectacles, contact lenses and intraocular lenses to correct astigmatism or to provide a range of focusing power from near to far; see also **cylinder, spherical lens** and **toric lens**

aspiration in ophthalmic usage, suction applied by a surgical instrument, usually to remove fluid or particulate matter from the eye; see also **irrigation and aspiration**

aspiration flow rate in phacoemulsification, the instrument setting that determines the maximum amount of fluid per unit of time (usually described in cubic centimeters per minute) that will flow through the eye into the instrument handpiece

asteroid hyalosis appearance of small white bodies in the vitreous humor, occurring most often in one eye, in the elderly and in males more than females, usually with little effect on vision

asthenopia impairment of function such that the eye is weak and/or tires easily, possibly accompanied by ocular pain, diminished vision and/or headache; **accommodative a.** asthenopia resulting from prolonged periods of accommodation (during reading or close work); **muscular a.** asthenopia attributable to tiring of the external ocular muscles; **nervous a.** asthenopia resulting from neurosis, characterized by eye fatigue and possibly constriction of the visual field; **tarsal a.** asthenopia attributable to pressure of the eyelids on the eye, which induces astigmatism

astigmatic clock vision test target consisting of straight radial lines (like the spokes of a wheel); the test subject looks at the center of the target and reports distortion of the lines, which will appear to be blurred along the axis of any astigmatism that might be present

astigmatism visual defect attributable to the presence of an elliptical (that is, egg- or football-shaped) rather than spherical shape in the refracting surfaces of the eye, resulting in the diffusion of light rays along a particular line in the visual field; an imaginary line drawn across the eye in its more nearly spherical area is called the steep axis and a line drawn across the more nearly cylindrical area is called the flat axis; **acquired a.** astigmatism resulting from some injury or insult to the eye; **against-the-rule a.** astigmatism in which the steep axis is within 30° of the horizontal (compare **with-the-rule a.**); **asymmetrical a.** astigmatism in which the steepest or flattest meridians in opposite halves of the eye do not lie on a straight line through the center of the eye; **complex a.** combination of corneal and lenticular astigmatism in the same eye; **compound a.** astigmatism in which the flat and steep axes are either both hyperopic (compound hyperopic a.) or myopic (compound myopic a.); **corneal a.** astigmatism attributable to the shape of the refractive surfaces of the cornea; **direct a.** see **with-the-rule a.; hypermetropic** or **hyperopic a.** astigmatism occurring in an eye that is hyperopic; **inverse a.** see **against-the-rule a.; irregular a.** astigmatism in which the flat and steep axes are not at right angles or astigmatism resulting from variable curvature along a given meridian of the eye; **lenticular a.** astigmatism attributable to the shape of the refractive surfaces of the crystalline lens; **mixed a.** astigmatism in which one axis is hyperopic and the other is myopic; **myopic a.** astigmatism occurring in an eye that is myopic; **oblique a.** astigmatism occurring along the 45° or 135° meridians (compare **against-the-rule a.** and **with-the-rule a.**); **pathological a.** astigmatism that results from some disease; **physiologic a.** small degree of astigmatism occurring normally in virtually all eyes, usually unnoticed; **regular a.** astigmatism in which the curvatures of the flat and steep axes are uniform across the width of the eye and lie approximately at right angles to each other; **simple a.** astigmatism occurring in an eye that is hyperopic (simple hyperopic a.) or myopic (simple myopic a.) along one axis and emmetropic along the axis 90° away; **symmetrical a.** astigmatism in which the steepest and flattest meridians in opposite halves of the eye lie on a straight line through the center of the eye; **with-the-rule a.** astigmatism in which the steep axis is within 30° of the vertical (so named because it is the most common type of astigmatism found in the human eye); compare **against-the-rule a.**

astigmia see **astigmatism**

atonic general term for lack of muscle tone

atonic ectropion condition in which weakness of the eyelid muscles results in the lid turning outward from the eye, exposing the conjunctiva

atopia general term for condition marked by unusually high allergic sensitivity of many tissues throughout the body to a number of allergens

atopic conjunctivitis see **conjunctivitis**

atresia iridis absence or severe diminution of the pupil at birth

attention reflex of the pupil change in size of pupil consequent to fixation of gaze upon an object

audito-oculogyric reflex turning of the eye in the direction of startling noises

autokeratoplasty keratoplasty in which only the patient's own corneal tissues are used

automated perimetry see **perimetry**

automated refractometry see **refractometry**

automated vitrectomy see **vitrectomy**

autorefractor instrument for measuring the refractive power of the eye that allows the patient to adjust various controls until clear vision is obtained

auxiometer or **auxometer** instrument that measures the magnifying power of lenses

axial hyperopia see **hyperopia**

axial length of the eye distance from the front of the cornea to the front of the retina along the principal axis of the eye

axial myopia see **myopia**

axis general term for imaginary line passing through a solid body, representing a hypothetical axis around which the object could be rotated; any one of several standard reference lines used to describe the anatomy and optical system of the eye, specifically: **external a.** axis from anterior pole of the eye to the posterior pole; **internal a.** axis from the anterior pole of the eye to the point on the retina just opposite the posterior pole; **lens a.** axis from the anterior pole to the posterior pole of the crystalline lens; **optical a.** axis passing through the optical center of the eye and perpendicular to the plane of the crystalline lens; **principal a.** see **optical a; pupillary a.** axis centered on and perpendicular to the plane of the pupil; **visual a.** axis along which light rays travel from an object to the macula (commonly referred to as the line of sight)

Bb

bacillary layer layer of column-like cells (rods and cones) in the retina

back surface toric see **posterior toric**

back vertex power portion of the total refractive power imparted by the rear surface of a lens; compare **front vertex power**

bacterial conjunctivitis see **conjunctivitis**

bacterial endophthalmitis see **endophthalmitis**

bag see **capsule**

Bagolini lens lens with fine parallel lines across its width, used in various vision tests

balanced salt solution mixture of water and salts (added to prevent electrolyte imbalance) used as an irrigating fluid in surgery

ballast see **prism ballast**

bandage contact lens see **contact lens**

band keratopathy or **keratitis** see **keratopathy**

Bard's sign phenomenon used to distinguish various types of nystagmus; patient with nystagmus is directed to follow finger motion across the field of view; in congenital nystagmus the rapid eye motions will decrease as the gaze shifts, while in organic nystagmus the motions increase

Barraquer keratomileusis see **keratomileusis**

bar reader device placed before the test subject to block out different portions of a page for each eye

barrel distortion image distortion that results from the steep curvature of spectacle lenses used to correct severe nearsightedness

Barre's sign impairment of iris reflex noted in patients with more generalized impairment of mental function

base curve general term for the curvature of the standard surface of a lens by which it is described; in spectacle and contact lenses, the base curve is measured on the less steep surface, most commonly the surface of the lens nearest the eye

base-down, base-in, base-out and **base-up prism** see **prism**

basement membrane general medical term for layer of tissue underlying some epithelial cell layers

basement membrane of choroid see **Bruch's membrane**

basement membrane of corneal epithelium thin membrane lying above Bowman's membrane to which the corneal epithelium adheres

beam splitter optical device that uses a partially reflective mirror to divide light into two beams similar in appearance but of reduced intensity, typically to create two images for viewing or two laser beams for delivery

bedewing (pronounced be-doo-ing) appearance of dew-like deposits on the cornea (which is said to be "bedewed"); see **guttata**

Behr pupil dilation of pupil resulting from a lesion far along the path of the optic nerve; because the two optic nerves cross, the dilated pupil will be on the opposite side of the body from the lesion

Bell palsy paralysis of the muscles of one side of the face due to inflammation of the facial nerve, resulting in an inability of the eyelids on that side to close completely

Bell phenomenon normal outward and upward rotation of the eyes that occurs when the lids are closed

benzalkonium chloride preservative often used in contact lens care solutions and topical ophthalmic medications

Berlin edema severe swelling of the macula following a blow to the head and resulting in permanent loss of part of the visual field (also known as **commotio retinae**)

Berry circle vision test target used to test stereopsis

best corrected visual acuity maximum visual acuity that can be achieved using corrective lenses to compensate for any refractive error (abbreviation: BCVA); see also **corrected visual acuity**; compare **uncorrected visual acuity**

best uncorrected visual acuity maximum visual acuity that is achieved without any corrective lenses (abbreviation: BUVA); compare **best corrected visual acuity**

biconcave lens lens that is concave (hollow like a bowl) on both surfaces (also called a **minus lens**)

biconvex lens lens that is convex (bulging outward) on both surfaces (also called a **plus lens**)

bifocal lens lens with two principal focal lengths (see also **multifocal lens**); a variety of such optical systems have been invented for vision correction: for example, bifocal spectacles used to correct presbyopia; there have also been bifocal contact lenses and bifocal intraocular lenses, but these represent only a small portion of the lenses in use or have not progressed beyond clinical trials

bifoveal fixation see **fixation**

bilateral anatomic term describing something that appears or occurs on both sides or, in its specific ophthalmic use, both eyes of an individual; compare **monocular**

binocular said of visual properties or processes that involve both eyes working together; compare **monocular**; for **binocular diplopia, binocular fixation** and **binocular fusion,** see definitions under main words

binocular microscope one that has two oculars (eyepieces) for both the viewer's eyes, thus providing a three-dimensional view

binocular ophthalmoscope see **ophthalmoscope**

binocular stereopsis or **vision** three-dimensional vision

biomicroscope see **slit lamp**

bioptics spectacles incorporating a telescopic lens system for use by low-vision patients

bipolar cells retinal cells that bridge the light-perceiving bacillary layer and underlying nerve cells

bitoric lens contact lens that has a toric front surface to correct astigmatism and a toric back surface to prevent the lens from rotating and keep it oriented to correct astigmatism in the proper axis

Bjerrum scotoma or **sign** visual field defect that extends in an arc from the physiologic blind spot around the center of the field of view; resulting from glaucoma and appearing as a deterioration from Seidel's scotoma

black cataract see **cataract**

blanching of sclera whitening of the sclera

blank unfinished spectacle or contact lens that does not yet exhibit its final refractive power

bleb soft-tissue space filled with fluid, most commonly in ophthalmic usage referring to a space created to receive drainage of aqueous fluid in glaucoma filtering surgery

blephar-, -o- combining form meaning *eyelid*

blepharitis inflammation of the eyelid, most often referring to the edge of the lid along which the eyelashes are located

blepharoconjunctivitis inflammation of the conjunctiva and eyelid

blepharophimosis condition in which the space between the eyelids is abnormally narrow

blepharoplasty general term for plastic surgical procedure of the eyelid(s) that can be reconstructive or cosmetic

blepharoplegia paralysis of the eyelids

blepharoptosis see **ptosis**

blepharorrhaphy suturing the eyelids together; also called **tarsorrhaphy**

blepharospasm uncontrollable muscle spasm that shuts the eye; **essential b.** that which is not attributable to any defect of the structures of the eye or nerves

blindness partial (as in the following terms) or total lack of the visual sense, more properly referred to as *amaurosis;* **color b.** colloquial term for impaired visual function at certain wavelengths of light (see also **achromatopsia** and **monochromatism**); **legal b.** state of visual impairment defined by public law or legal contract (for example, an insurance policy) precluding certain activities such as driving and qualifying individuals for certain tax or social service benefits; legal blindness is usually defined as Snellen acuity of 20/200 or less in the better-seeing eye or remaining visual field of 20° or less; **night b.** see **nyctalopia; river b.** see **onchocerciasis; word b.** see **alexia;** see also **count-finger vision, hand-motion vision, light perception vision, no light perception vision** and **visual acuity**

blind spot area where the retina is joined to the optic nerve such that it forms a "funnel" of nerve cells that is not sensitive to light in its center; not usually noticed subjectively but readily detected even with the most simple visual field test; more properly called the *physiologic blind spot* to distinguish it from damaged areas of the retina; see also **scotoma**

blink reflex automatic response of eyelids to close when the cornea is touched

blood-aqueous barrier, blood-eye barrier or **blood-vitreous barrier** physiologic mechanisms that generally prevent passage of fluid or cells from the blood into the eye

blowout fracture of the orbit fracture in which the bones comprising the eye socket are disconnected and displaced outward from their normal position, usually with massive damage to the soft tissues of the eyeball

blue-yellow perimetry colloquial term for visual field test in which the test targets are blue and yellow, which appears to enhance the ability of the test to locate field defects

blur circle see **conoid of Sturm**

blur point in testing visual acuity, the blur point is reached when the refractive power of a lens or prism can no longer be increased without causing vision to be blurred

boric acid substance once used widely as an eyewash ingredient

botulin or **botulinum** toxic substance produced by *Clostridium botulinum* bacteria used for treatment of blepharospasm and certain types of strabismus

Bowman's capsule, layer or **membrane** outermost layer of the cornea lying above the corneal stroma and beneath the corneal epithelium

branch retinal artery one of the small arteries that branch off the central retinal artery

branch retinal artery occlusion blockage of a branch retinal artery, usually in the temporal retina, impairing retinal blood flow but usually resulting in no loss of vision or only minor visual field loss

branch retinal vein one of the small veins in the retina that drain into the central retinal vein

branch retinal vein occlusion blockage of blood flow in an area where a branch retinal vein is crossed by a branch retinal artery, resulting in retinal hemorrhage and a sudden blurring or loss of vision in part of the visual field

break-up time length of time from the blink of an eye until the tear film evaporates, usually measured at the slit lamp using fluorescein dye staining

bridle suture suture placed through the insertion of an extraocular muscle in order to give the surgeon control over the position of the eye

Brown syndrome condition, usually congenital but possibly as a result of arthritis, in which the tendon sheath of the superior oblique muscle does not relax and thus prevents the eye from looking upward

Bruch's membrane innermost layer of the choroid on which the retinal pigment epithelium adheres

brunescent brown; descriptive of very mature, dark cataracts

B-scan as used in ophthalmology, an ultrasound examination to create a cross-sectional view of the eye

buckling procedure see **scleral buckling procedure**

bulb in ophthalmic usage, synonym for the eyeball

bulbar conjunctiva portion of the conjunctiva that covers the eyeball, extending almost to the corneoscleral limbus; compare **palpebral conjunctiva**

bullous keratopathy degeneration of cornea; **pseudophakic b.k.** corneal degeneration attributable and consequent to implantation of an intraocular lens

buphthalmia, -os condition in which the eye is abnormally large, most often used to describe pediatric eyes in which high intraocular pressure has distended the globe

Cc

caloric nystagmus see **nystagmus**

canaliculus tear duct, more properly called canaliculus nasolacrimalis; plural: canaliculi

canal of Schlemm see **Schlemm's canal**

candela standard unit used in measurement of the intensity of light; the metric unit that replaced the candle; abbreviation: cd

cannula tube used in surgery to perform irrigation or aspiration of fluids or to introduce smaller instruments into an incision

can-opener capsulotomy surgical technique in which a series of small cuts are made in a circle around the periphery of the anterior lens capsule, which is then removed; compare **capsulorrhexis**

canthotomy surgical procedure in which an incision is made into the area where the upper and lower eyelids meet

canthus either of two angles formed by the meeting of the upper and lower eyelids; the one near the temple is called the **lateral canthus** and the one near the nose is called the **medial canthus**; plural: canthi

capsular advancement see **advancement**

capsular opacification cloudiness of the lens capsule resulting from the spread of lens epithelial cells across the part of the capsule that remains after cataract extraction

capsule general medical term for the outer membrane surrounding an anatomic structure, most commonly in ophthalmic usage referring to the **lens capsule,** the transparent round sac containing the lens of the eye, attached at its periphery by the zonules to the ciliary body, often referred to as the capsular bag or simply "the bag;" **anterior c.** front portion of the capsule between the lens and the iris; **posterior c.** rear portion of the capsule between the lens and the vitreous body; **Tenon's c.** thin, outermost membrane of the eye, enclosing the entire globe except for the cornea

capsulectomy general term for surgical removal of a capsule

capsulorrhexis 1. surgical procedure in which an anterior capsulotomy is made by puncturing, then grasping and tearing a hole in the capsule rather than by simply cutting it with a sharp instrument; 2. the opening made in the capsule in this manner

capsulotomy 1. surgical procedure to make an opening in a capsule, usually the lens capsule as the first step in extracapsular cataract extraction; 2. the opening made in the capsule in this manner; **anterior c.** surgical procedure to open the anterior capsule (or the opening itself), most commonly as one step in removal of a cataractous lens (see also **can-opener c.** and **capsulorrhexis**); **posterior c.** surgical procedure to open the posterior capsule (or the opening itself), often referring to the procedure performed with the Nd:YAG laser to open an opacified posterior capsule months or years after cataract extraction

carbon dioxide laser see **laser**

cardinal points six points on the axis of an optical system that are used in describing its properties

cardinal positions of gaze six directions to which test subjects are told to direct their eyes so that the coordinated function of the extraocular yoke muscles can be assessed: right, left, up and to the right, down and to the right, up and to the left, down and to the left

caruncle see **lacrimal caruncle**

cataphoria turning of the eyes downward immediately following the cessation of visual stimuli

cataract area of opacification in ocular tissue that impedes the transmission of light rays to the retina; most commonly, the opacification of the lens that occurs as a natural consequence of aging, which is a leading cause of blindness in many parts of the world but surgically corrected on a wide scale (and with great success) in the developed world where ophthalmologic care is available; **after c.** opacification, usually of the posterior lens capsule, following removal of a cataractous crystalline lens; **annular c.** ring-shaped opacity of the lens in which the central lens remains clear; **axial c.** opacity located in the optical axis of the crystalline lens; **black c.** very mature (that is, advanced stage) cataract that is opaque black, very dense and hard; **brunescent c.** very mature cataract that has a brownish appearance, often very dense and hard; **capsular c.** clouding of the lens capsule, typically by overgrowth of epithelial cells (as often happens after implantation of an intraocular lens); **congenital c.** cataract present at birth; **cortical c.** opacification of the lens cortex, usually in radial streaks or spokes, rather than the nucleus; **degenerative c.** opacification of ocular tissue that results from a degenerative change (compare **developmental c.**); **developmental c.** opacification of ocular tissue that results from a disturbance of normal development; **hypermature c.** progression of mature cataract to state in which the lens begins to shrink and eventually soften, with harmful leakage of lens proteins; **intumescent c.** opacified lens that has swelled up with absorbed fluid; **juvenile c.** cataract occurring in childhood; **lenticular c.** opacification of the crystalline lens; **mature c.** crystalline lens that has become opaque and exceedingly hard over a prolonged time; **morgagnian c.** progression of hypermature cataract in which the lens cortex is completely liquefied and the hard, opaque nucleus is no longer held stationary in the lens capsule; **nuclear c.** or **nuclear sclerotic c.** opacification of the crystalline lens; **peripheral c.** opacification that is out of the optical axis and thus only minimally impairs vision; **polar c.** opacification located at the anterior or posterior pole of the crystalline lens; **posterior subcapsular c.** opacification of the posterior part of the lens nucleus best viewed by retroillumination; **secondary c.** opacification of tissues other than the lens (of the lens capsule, for example) after previous surgery removing the crystalline lens; **senile c.** cataract occurring in an elderly individual as a natural part of aging; **subcapsular c.** opacification of the inner surfaces of the lens capsule caused by overgrowth of epithelial cells; **traumatic c.** opacification of ocular tissue (especially the crystalline lens) resulting from a blow or penetrating injury to the eye, often quite rapid in onset and profound in extent

cataract extraction general term for surgical procedures to remove the opacified crystalline lens of the eye; cataract extraction is essentially another term for crystalline lens removal, and all such procedures have in common an incision into the anterior chamber of the eye, but there are many variations in the size of the incision, its location and the instrumentation and technique used to remove the lens material; the eye immediately after cataract extraction is in a state known as aphakia (without a lens), and an eye in which an intraocular lens has been implanted is said to be pseudophakic ("false" lens); see also **cryoextraction, extracapsular cataract extraction, intracapsular cataract extraction** and **phacoemulsification**

cataractogenic causing or facilitating the formation of cataract

cataractous ocular tissue that is like or affected by cataract

cat's eye pupil condition in which the pupil is a narrow vertical slit

cavitation in ophthalmic usage, a phenomenon in which the ultrasonically vibrating phaco-emulsification tip creates microscopic areas of intense turbulence that pulverizes lens material

cell in ophthalmic usage, the appearance of white blood cells in the anterior chamber as a result of inflammation following surgery or trauma; see also **flare**

cell and flare in ophthalmic usage, usually the appearance of white blood cells in the anterior chamber accompanied by the presence of protein particles in the aqueous humor, indicating intraocular inflammation, usually after surgery or trauma

cellophane maculopathy see **epiretinal membrane**

central fixation see **fixation**

central fusion see **fusion**

central retinal artery one of the main blood vessels bringing blood into the retina from the ophthalmic artery

central retinal artery occlusion blockage of the central retinal artery, resulting in sudden, permanent loss of vision across a wide area of the visual field

central retinal vein major vein that drains blood from the retina, exiting the eye in the area of the optic nerve

central retinal vein occlusion blockage of the central retinal vein resulting in retinal hemorrhage and sudden loss of vision, usually involving the central visual field

central scotoma see **scotoma**

central serous chorioretinopathy condition similar to central serous retinopathy, except with greater involvement of the choroid

central serous retinopathy condition in which there is swelling and elevation of retinal tissues in the area of the macula, sometimes progressing to the point of detachment, that causes a perceptible but usually not permanent visual field loss

central suppression action of the brain to ignore the portion of the image in the center of the visual field

centrocecal scotoma see **scotoma**

chalazion cyst of the eyelid resulting from inflammation (see also **hordeolum** and **meibomian cyst**)

chatter in ophthalmic usage, undesirable phenomenon in phacoemulsification in which the crystalline lens rapidly vibrates on the instrument tip as it is simultaneously attracted by aspiration and repelled by the vibration of the tip

chemosis swelling of the conjunctiva; adjective: chemotic

chiasm general anatomic term for an intersection (from the Greek letter chi, X); see **optic chiasm**

choked disk see **papilledema**

chondroitin sulfate component of some viscoelastic materials

choriopathy noninflammatory disease of the choroid

chorioretinal of or involving the choroid and retina

choroid highly vascular tissue layer lying under the retina, merging at the angle of the anterior chamber with the ciliary body and iris (all three areas comprising the uvea)

choroidal detachment separation of the choroid from the sclera, usually as a result of injury

choroidal neovascularization condition in which new blood vessels grow into the choroid beneath the retinal pigment epithelium

choroidal neovascular membrane network of vascular tissue resulting from choroidal neovascularization

choroidal nevus small, well-defined area of benign pigmentation or vascularization in the choroid

choroideremia sex-linked hereditary condition in which the retinal pigment epithelium and choroid begin to degenerate in the first few months or years after birth, in males eventually leading to blindness but in females rarely causing significant vision loss

choroiditis inflammatory disease of the choroid

chromatic aberration uneven focusing of an optical system such that white light is partially or completely broken down into its component colors

chronic in medical usage, denoting the long-term or non-emergency (compare **acute**)

cicatrix scar tissue (adjective: cicatricial); some cases of ectropion and entropion are described as cicatricial, and some glaucoma operations construct what is known as a cicatricial filter

cilia plural of cilium

ciliaris see **ciliary muscle**

ciliary 1. of or related to the eyelashes; 2. of or related to the ring-shaped structure joining the iris and choroid, the primary producer of aqueous fluid

ciliary arteries several branches of the ophthalmic artery that carry blood to every anatomic structure of the eye except the inner part of the retina

ciliary body ring-shaped structure joining the iris to the choroid, containing the ciliary muscle and ciliary processes

ciliary muscle ring-shaped muscle in the ciliary body; it contracts upon near vision, resulting in accommodation

ciliary nerves any of several nerve fiber bundles that either carry nerve impulses to the pupillary sphincter and ciliary muscle, as well as carrying impulses from the cornea (short ciliary nerves), or carry impulses to the pupillary dilator muscle or sensory impulses from the cornea, iris and ciliary body (long ciliary nerves)

ciliary processes finger-shaped extensions of the ciliary body that produce aqueous humor and provide an attachment for the zonules that support the lens capsule

ciliary spasm prolonged contraction of the ciliary muscle due to some pathologic condition

ciliary sulcus groove formed by the junction of the ciliary body and iris; posterior chamber intraocular lenses are sometimes placed into the sulcus when implantation into the lens capsule is not possible

ciliary veins any of several veins that drain blood from the major anatomic structures of the eye

cilium term for the eyelid, the edge of the eyelid, or the eyelashes (plural: cilia)

circle of Zinn see **annulus of Zinn**

circumduction of the eye circular "rolling" of the eye, applicable to voluntary and involuntary movement

clear lensectomy refractive surgical procedure to correct large degrees of nearsightedness by removing the crystalline lens

clock dial see **astigmatic clock**

C-loop lens see **intraocular lens**

closed-angle glaucoma see **glaucoma**

CMV retinitis see **retinitis**

cobalt blue filter light filter placed on the slit lamp light source to induce fluorescence during fluorescein dye staining of the cornea

coherent light light in which all of the component waves are in phase; see also **laser**

collarette 1. encrusting of the base of an eyelash in blepharitis; 2. border between pupillary and ciliary zones of the iris, visible on the anterior surface of the iris as a line of transitional color about 1.5 mm from the edge of the pupil

collyrium general term for an eyewash

coloboma partial absence of or gap in ocular structures, as in retinal coloboma, iris coloboma, etc., usually in the lower half of the eye and usually a result of incomplete formation of fetal tissue; **atypical c.** coloboma in the upper half of the eye

color subjective perception of the varying wavelengths of light

color adaptation see **adaptation**

color blindness see **blindness** and **deuteranopia**

columnar layer cell layer of the retina consisting of column-like cells (rods and cones); also called the bacillary layer

comitant see **concomitant**

comitant strabismus see **strabismus**

commotio retinae see **Berlin edema**

compound astigmatism or **compound myopic astigmatism** see **astigmatism**

concave having a curved, indented surface, like the inside of a bowl; compare **convex**

concave lens lens with a concave surface, which causes parallel rays of light to diverge and thus can be used to correct myopia; see also **minus lens; double c. lens** lens that has two concave surfaces

concavoconvex lens lens that has one concave and one convex surface

conclination tendency for the eyes to point toward one another (rather than remaining parallel) when the gaze is directed upward or downward

concomitant adjective describing a constant, uniform relationship between the lines of sight of the two eyes that depends upon the direction of gaze, indicating normal extraocular muscle function; compare **incomitant**

concomitant strabismus see **strabismus**

cone geometric term used in ophthalmic applications to describe anatomic structures and optical properties; **distraction c.** white crescent-shaped area sometimes seen on funduscopy in myopic eyes; **myopic c.** staphyloma at the posterior pole of the eye; **ocular c.** the eyeball and its sheath of muscle, blood vessels and nerves, approximately conical in shape; **retinal cones** or **cone cells** one of two types of light-sensitive cells in the retina (rods are the other type); often simply referred to as cones, they are concentrated in the macula and function in the discrimination of fine detail in the field of view under bright light conditions

confrontation field test method for measuring the approximate extent of the visual field in which examiner sits facing the test subject and holds a target object far to the subject's side, then brings it slowly into the field of view; the subjects reports when the target object becomes visible

congruous similar in form

congruous field defect visual field defects of similar shape in both eyes

congruous hemianopia loss of half the visual field in each eye in which the field defects are the same size, shape and location

conjunctiva ocular tissue comprising the inner surface of the eyelids (**palpebral c.**), which folds in to join with the sclera (**bulbar c.**); the "pocket" of the fold is called the cul de sac; **limbal c.** edge of the conjunctiva overlying the sclera near its transition zone into the cornea

conjunctival injection condition in which the conjunctiva is red, swollen and engorged with dilated blood vessels

conjunctivitis general term for inflammation of the conjunctiva; colloquially known as pink eye; **allergic c.** conjunctivitis resulting from an allergic reaction, either to airborne allergens or substances (such as topical medications) placed into the eye; **atopic c.** conjunctivitis occurring as one manifestation of atopia, a condition of unusually high allergic sensitivity of many tissues throughout the body to a number of allergens; **bacterial c.** conjunctivitis resulting from an infection of the surface tissues of the eye; **follicular c.** appearance of tiny clear or yellow sacs of lymphocytes and inflammatory cells on the conjunctiva after prolonged irritation, often as a result of viral infection; **giant papillary c.** condition in which wart-like protrusions (papillae) appear on the inside of the eyelid accompanied by mucous discharge; **herpetic c.** conjunctivitis resulting from an infection with herpes virus; **inclusion c.**

inflammation of the conjunctiva due to presence of chlamydia organisms; **vernal c.** chronic allergic conjunctivitis that occurs in both eyes during warm weather

conoid of Sturm geometric representation of light refracted through a lens that is spherical along one axis and cylindrical along another

consecutive in ophthalmic usage, describing a condition (usually unwanted) that results after surgery (for example, consecutive hyperopia is an adverse result of radial keratotomy to correct myopia)

consensual papillary reflex phenomenon in which both pupils constrict when either one is stimulated by light or accommodation; its absence is an indication of some disorder of the ocular nervous system

constant esotropia see **esotropia**

constant exotropia see **exotropia**

contact angle see **wetting angle**

contact lens 1. vision-correcting lens placed directly on the cornea of the eye; composed of polymethylmethacrylate (**hard c.l.**) when modern contact lenses were introduced in the 1950s, contact lenses currently are made from silicone or water-containing hydroxyethyl-methacrylate (**soft c.l.**) or polymers formulated to transmit oxygen (**gas-permeable c.l.**); **bandage c.l.** lens used for therapeutic purposes (usually to protect the cornea or deliver medication following surgery or trauma) rather than to correct vision; **corneal c.l.** contact lens designed to rest upon the cornea rather than extending onto the sclera; **fenestrated c.l.** contact lens perforated with one or more holes in order to allow air or tear fluid to penetrate through the lens to the eye; **fitting c.l.** lens used to check for correct fit on patient before a contact lens prescription is written; **haptic c.l.** see **scleral c.l.; scleral c.l.** contact lens designed so that its periphery rests on the sclera rather than the cornea; **trial c.l.** see **fitting c.l.;** see also **aspheric lens, bifocal lens, multifocal lens** and **toric lens**; 2. hand-held lens system, usually incorporating prisms and/or mirrors, placed on the cornea to provide a view inside the eye or to focus laser energy for delivery into the eye

contrast property of an image such that it has bright and dark areas; the relative brightness of the various components can be measured in comparison to each other or against a reference gray scale

contrast sensitivity ability to distinguish fine gradations of brightness, often diminished under conditions of glare (as in cases of cataract or uncorrected astigmatism)

convergence 1. in optics, the gathering together of parallel light rays to a point of focus after passing through a plus lens; 2. in ophthalmic usage, coordinated action of ocular muscles that draws both eyes inward to fixate upon the same point in space (also called **positive convergence**); the processes of convergence and accommodation normally are linked; **accommodative c.** convergence stimulated by and working in conjunction with accommodation; **far point of c.** imaginary point at which the visual axes cross when both eyes are fixated at infinity (also called *minimum convergence*); **fusional c.** convergence operating to keep an image focused upon the foveae of both eyes; **near point of c.** imaginary point at which the visual axes cross when the eyes are fixated on as near an object as possible (also called *maximum convergence*); **negative c.** see **divergence**; **positive c.** synonym for convergence; **tonic c.** degree of convergence maintained by the tone of the ocular muscles, bringing the eyes inward from the divergent angle at which they are positioned in the orbits

convergence insufficiency acquired condition in which the eyes fail to turn inward enough to achieve fusion during near vision

convergent lens see **plus lens**

convergent strabismus see **esotropia**

convex having a rounded, protruding surface, like a globe; compare **concave**

convex lens lens with a convex surface, which causes parallel rays of light to converge and thus can be used to correct hyperopia; see also **plus lens; double c. lens** lens that has two convex surfaces

convexoconcave lens lens that has one convex and one concave surface

core-, -a- combining form meaning *pupil*

corectopia condition in which the pupil is not in the center of the iris

cornea clear structure at the front, central part of the eye imparting the greatest focusing power of all the ocular media, composed (from outer- to innermost) of the epithelium, Bowman's membrane, the stroma, Descemet's membrane and the endothelium; the cornea is continuous with the sclera and consists of similar tough, fibrous tissue; see also words beginning with the root **kerat-,** meaning *cornea*

corneal abrasion injury in which tissues are scraped from an area on the surface of the cornea, usually involving the corneal epithelium but possibly extending more deeply

corneal astigmatism see **astigmatism**

corneal bedewing appearance of cornea in which dew-like beads are seen on the surface of the cornea, usually visible only under magnification

corneal button piece of corneal tissue, either full-thickness (for penetrating keratoplasty) or partial thickness (a lamellar keratoplasty), intended for use as a graft

corneal decompensation condition in which chronic failure of the corneal endothelium to maintain the proper water content of the corneal stroma results in swelling, clouding and degeneration of the cornea

corneal dellen small concavities at the outer edges of the cornea that sometimes appear after ocular surgery

corneal dystrophy general term for hereditary condition, defective development or degeneration of corneal tissue; **endothelial c.d.** condition, possibly worse in one eye than the other but always present bilaterally, in which black spheres appear in the corneal endothelium, eventually resulting in loss of vision due to corneal edema as normal endothelial function is impaired (see also **guttata**); **fingerprint c.d.** condition in which small concentric lines with the appearance of a fingerprint appear in the corneal epithelium; **Fuchs d.** progressive degeneration of the cornea related to dysfunction of the corneal epithelium

corneal ectasia bulging outward of the cornea that occurs when corneal tissue is thinned or weakened

corneal edema condition in which the cornea swells with water and becomes cloudy; almost always a result of damage to the corneal endothelium

corneal endothelium innermost layer of the cornea, only one cell thick, which acts to pump excess water out of the cornea; these cells are quite delicate and do not regenerate if damaged

corneal epithelium outermost layer of the cornea, only one cell thick, which regenerates rapidly if damaged or even if (as is done in certain ophthalmic procedures) the whole layer is removed

corneal erosion loss of the corneal epithelium over some or all of the area of the cornea; **recurrent c.e.** chronic condition in which corneal erosion periodically occurs due to inadequate adhesion of the epithelium to its basement membrane

cornea guttata see **guttata** and **endothelial corneal dystrophy** under **corneal dystrophy**

corneal hydrops accumulation of aqueous fluid within the cornea as a result of the loss of tissue integrity of the corneal endothelium and Descemet's membrane

corneal lathing see **keratomileusis**

corneal map see **corneal topography**

corneal melting condition in which layers of the cornea degenerate and slough off due to an inflammatory process

corneal reflex see **blink reflex**

corneal stroma transparent connective tissue making up the main body of the cornea

corneal topography imaging technique in which an image projected onto the cornea is analyzed by a computer to obtain a representation of the shape of the corneal surface and thus an indication of its refractive power; also known as videokeratography

corneal transplant see **keratoplasty**

corneal ulcer loss of tissue from the surface of the cornea due to a disease process, often an infection

corneoscleral of or involving the cornea and sclera

corneoscleral junction or **spur** see **scleral spur**

corrected visual acuity visual acuity measured with corrective lenses in place (abbreviation: VA_{cc}); see also **best corrected visual acuity** and **uncorrected visual acuity**

correction in ophthalmic usage, spectacles or contact lenses prescribed to counteract myopia, hyperopia, astigmatism or any other ametropia

correspondence see **retinal correspondence**

cortex in ophthalmic usage, the soft outer portion of the crystalline lens of the eye

cortical attachments areas in which the nucleus and cortex of the crystalline lens adhere together

cotton-wool spots small areas of the retinal nerve fiber layer that have lost their blood supply and become wispy white areas with no clear borders; see also **retinal exudates**

couching obsolete treatment for cataract in which the whole lens of the eye was detached and pushed out of the visual axis, usually accomplished with a needle inserted into the anterior chamber of the eye

count-finger vision very low level of visual acuity in which no greater detail can be perceived than the number of fingers held before the eyes; see also **hand-motion vision, light perception vision, no light perception vision** and **visual acuity**

cover test test to determine presence of phoria or tropia by having the subject fixate on a target while the examiner covers first one eye, then the other with an occluder, observing any movement of the uncovered eye; if there is no movement of the eye, the patient is orthophoric; movement of the eye in the same direction that the occluder moves indicates exophoria, movement in the opposite direction indicates esophoria and downward movement of the eye indicates hyperphoria in the eye that had been covered; the cover test may be performed while holding prisms in front of the eye to determine how much prismatic power is needed to neutralize the movement; **alternate c.t.** cover test performed by quickly moving the occluder from one eye to the other so that there is no time for binocular fixation to occur

cover-uncover test cover test performed on one eye only

crazing in ophthalmic usage, the appearance of a network of fine lines or cracks on a lens, most often a contact lens covered by some type of plaque

cribriform plate see **lamina cribrosa**

cribrosa see **lamina cribrosa**

cross cylinder lens comprising two cylindrical components of the same power, one plus and one minus, superimposed at right angles to each other, used to identify the presence of astigmatism; see also **Jackson cross cylinder lens**

crossed diplopia see **heteronymous diplopia**

cross fixation condition in which the left eye becomes dominant in gaze toward the extreme right and the right eye becomes dominant in gaze toward the extreme left

cryo- combining form meaning *cold,* used in medical terminology to describe treatments or surgical procedures involving very low temperatures (usually several hundred degrees below zero)

cryoextraction technique of intracapsular cataract extraction in which the lens capsule and its contents are frozen to the tip of a surgical instrument (cryoprobe) and removed as a unit; now largely abandoned in the U.S. in favor of extracapsular cataract extraction but still performed by many surgeons around the world; see also **cataract extraction, extracapsular cataract extraction, intra-capsular cataract extraction** and **phaco-emulsification**

cryopexy surgical procedure that attempts to fix a tissue into place (most commonly in ophthalmic usage, a detached retina against the choroid) by application of extreme cold

cryophake instrument used in cataract cryoextraction

cryoprobe general term for instrument used in cryosurgery

cryoretinopexy see **retinopexy**

cryosurgery or **cryotherapy** general terms for application of extreme cold to tissue

crystalline lens proper term for the natural lens of the eye (usually called simply "the lens"), consisting of a soft outer cortex and hard nucleus in the center; use of the full term *crystalline lens* is helpful as a distinction from artificial lenses manufactured for vision correction

cul de sac general anatomic term for a sac with only one opening (from French for "bottom of the bag"); in ophthalmic usage, the sac formed by the bulbar and palpebral conjunctivae; see also **conjunctiva**

cup in ophthalmic usage, sign of glaucomatous damage in which the optic disk is affected by an area of concavity, representing nonfunctioning retinal cells

cupping property of the optic disk such that a cup (see above) is present

cup-to-disk ratio measure of the proportion of damaged area (cup) to visually functional area (disk) of the retina, representing the relative progression of glaucomatous damage; see also **glaucoma**

cycl-, -o- combining form meaning *circle* or *ring;* in ophthalmic usage, the iris and/or ciliary body

cyclitic membrane formation of fibrous tissue in the anterior part of the vitreous body as a result of severe inflammation of the ciliary body

cyclitis inflammation of the ciliary body

cyclocryotherapy application of very low temperatures to the ciliary body; performed in an attempt to decrease the production of aqueous fluid by the ciliary processes as a treatment for glaucoma

cyclodestruction general term for glaucoma surgical procedures that destroy portions of the ciliary body (as with extreme cold, laser energy or other means) in order to decrease the production of aqueous fluid

cyclodialysis largely abandoned glaucoma surgical procedure in which the root of the iris is detached from the ciliary body so that aqueous fluid may pass more easily out of the anterior chamber and thus reduce intraocular pressure

cycloduction rotation or "rolling" of the eyes

cycloplegia paralysis of the ciliary muscle in which the eye does not accommodate in response to the usual stimuli

cylinder 1. in optics, a lens that is flat along one axis and circularly curved along the perpendicular axis, making a cylindrical shape, or the property of a lens that is relatively flat along one axis and more circular along the perpendicular axis; 2. in refraction, the component of refractive error that can be corrected with a cylindrical lens (roughly synonymous with *astigmatism*); compare **sphere; minus c.** refracting surface of a lens in which the lens material is fashioned into the concave reverse of a cylindrical shape (that is, as if a cylinder had been carved out of the lens and discarded); **plus c.** refracting surface of a lens in which the lens material is fashioned into the convex shape of a cylinder

cystoid macular edema swelling of the central focusing area of the retina, typically as a result of trauma and often as a complication of ophthalmic surgery

cystotome surgical instrument for cutting a sac; most often in ophthalmic usage, instrument for cutting into the lens capsule

cytomegalovirus retinitis see **retinitis**

Dd

dacry-, -o- combining form meaning *tear fluid;* see also combining forms beginning with **lacri-**

dacryocyst sac adjacent to the eye that holds tears

dacryocystorhinostomy procedure in which an opening between the dacryocyst and the nasal passage is created or reopened; abbreviation: DCR

dark adaptation see **adaptation**

decentration general term for misalignment; in ophthalmic usage, usually referring to displacement of a lens (particularly an intraocular lens) out of the visual axis

decussation general anatomic term for an intersection; **optic nerve d.** see **chiasm**

degenerative cataract see **cataract**

degenerative myopia see **myopia**

dehiscence general medical term for a splitting open of tissue, often as a result of fibrosis in the course of healing of a traumatic or surgical wound, typically in ophthalmic usage referring to splitting of retinal tissue or breakage of the lens zonular fibers

dellen see **corneal dellen**

dendritic describing a tree-like shape; used often in ophthalmic terminology to describe lesions on the cornea that have a branched appearance (as in *dendritic keratitis,* for example)

depth of field space in front of and behind an object upon which the eyes are fixated, in which other objects can be seen clearly; the depth of field is typically very shallow for nearby objects, and for very distant objects there is usually a very deep depth of field

depth perception ability to discern the relative distance of objects within the field of view, made possible by the varying degrees of convergence necessary to focus upon objects at varying distances from the observer

dermatochalasis condition in which a redundant flap of skin overlaps the eyelid and presses the lashes inward

Descemet's membrane inner tissue layer of the cornea on which the corneal endothelium adheres

detachment separation of tissue layers that are normally attached; in ophthalmic usage, most commonly referring to the retina or choroid; see also **retinal detachment**

deuteranopia, -opsia retinal pigment deficiency resulting in the inability to distinguish shades of red or green; this is the most common form of "color blindness"

deviation in ophthalmic usage, a turning of the eye from the point of fixation; **convergent d.** see **esotropia; dissociated vertical d.** deviation of an eye upward when it is occluded and the other eye is fixating; **divergent d.** see **exotropia; primary d.** deviation of the eye that normally does not fixate in strabismus when the other eye is fixating; **secondary d.**

deviation of the eye that normally fixates in strabismus when the eye that normally does not fixate is forced to do so; **skew d.** condition in which the eyes move in opposite directions (for example, one eye moves upward when the fellow eye is directed downward)

dextro- prefix describing structures or processes appearing or occurring toward the right; referring to the right eye in ophthalmic usage, as in the phrase *oculus dexter;* compare **sinistro-**

diabetic retinopathy ocular effect of the systemic disorder, diabetes mellitus; characterized by edema and neovascularization of the retina, with progressive loss of vision if left untreated; laser therapy is currently applied in cases of diabetic retinopathy

dialysis in ophthalmic usage, the separation of connected tissues or structures

diffraction property of light attributable to its wave-like nature; light passing through a very narrow opening (about the same width as the wavelength of the light) is bent from its original path; theoretically, diffraction provides an alternative optical system to refraction for artificial lens design

diffractive multifocal lens optical system that attempts to use diffraction in order to impart two or more focal points to incoming light, one "fundamental" focus provided by conventional refractive optics and the other(s) provided by diffraction; diffractive multifocal contact lenses and diffractive multifocal intraocular lenses have been manufactured and tested in humans

diffuse illumination in slit lamp biomicroscopy, use of non-focused, scattered light to provide a view of the whole eye and its adnexa, often for photography

diffuser filter for the light source of an optical instrument that scatters light without changing its color, thereby reducing reflections that can occur with point sources of illumination

digital tonometry method for estimating intraocular pressure by judging the eyeball's resistance to a finger pressed against it

dilation or **dilatation** general term for widening of an opening; in ophthalmic usage, the widening of the pupil in dim light or as a result of pharmaceuticals (more properly called mydriasis); dilation must be induced in order to perform certain intraocular examinations and surgical procedures

dimer substance composed of two components; see also **excimer laser** under **laser**

diode laser see **laser**

diopter 1. measure of the focusing power of a lens, defined as the reciprocal of the focal length measured in meters; abbreviation: D; for example, a lens that focuses light from a very distant object ("infinity") to a point 1 m behind the lens has a power of 1 D, whereas a lens that focused light at 2 m has a power of 0.5 D; 2. by analogy, degrees of myopia (designated as minus diopters) or hyperopia (designated as plus diopters), as well as astigmatism, are described by the dioptric power of the lens prescribed to correct the defect (resulting in descriptions like "the patient is a four diopter myope"); see also **prism diopter**

dioptric adjectival form of diopter

diplopia perception of two images where there is only one object (colloquially known as double vision); **binocular d.** double vision resulting from the lack of fusion of the images from each eye; **crossed d.** double vision in which the image from one eye is seen on the opposite side of the image from the fellow eye; **monocular d.** double image seen when only one eye is used, resulting from some abnormality of the ocular media, the presence of a prism or a neurological problem in processing the image from the retina; **vertical d.** double vision in which the two images are seen one above the other

direct illumination in slit lamp biomicroscopy, method of viewing by shining light from the slit lamp light source upon the ocular structures to be viewed; compare **indirect illumination**

direct ophthalmoscopy process of viewing the internal structures of the eye at close range through instrumentation that presents the right-side-up, unreversed image of the interior of the eye; most often referring to the use of a hand-held ophthalmoscope through which the examiner looks with one eye (thus obtaining only a two-dimensional image with no depth); compare **indirect ophthalmoscopy**

disciform keratitis see **keratitis**

disk or, less preferred, **disc** general anatomic term for flat, circular structures; in ophthalmic usage, portion of the retina where nerve fibers converge to form the optic nerve (more properly called the optic disk or the optic nerve head)

disk drusen see **drusen**

dispensing in ophthalmic usage, the business of selling spectacles and/or contact lenses as well as prescribing them, usually combined with a description of the practitioner (for example, a "dispensing optometrist")

dissociated vertical deviation see **deviation**

distance vision vision of objects relatively far from the eye, approaching infinity; the distance at which visual tasks such as driving are considered to be performed, generally defined to be a minimum of about 20 feet; compare **near vision**

divergence 1. in optics, the spreading outward of parallel light rays after passing through a minus lens; 2. outward turning of one or both eyes; compare **convergence**

divergent lens see **minus lens**

divergent strabismus see **strabismus**

Dk unit of measure of the oxygen transmission of contact lens materials, given as the product of the material's oxygen diffusion coefficient (D) times oxygen solubility (k) in the material at a given thickness, temperature and hydration

doll's eye sign turning of the eyes in the opposite direction from which the head is moved

dominant eye the eye that is subjectively preferred for use by an individual, much like the way one hand or the other is preferred; compare **nondominant eye**

Donders law for any given direction of gaze and head position, the extraocular muscles exert the same torsion, regardless of how the eye was moved to attain the direction of gaze

Doppler ultrasound imaging technique in which the reflection of high-frequency sound waves from a moving object are analyzed to create a representation of the movement; used in ophthalmic applications to study ocular blood flow, especially in the retina

dot-and-blot hemorrhage appearance of small hemorrhages in the tissues of the retina, usually associated with diabetic retinopathy but also seen with other conditions

double concave lens see **concave lens**

double convex lens see **convex lens**

double vision see **diplopia**

drusen small, circular, light-colored bodies that appear on the optic disk as a normal consequence of aging or in some disease processes; see also **retinal exudates**

dry eye syndrome common condition in which a defect in the composition of the tears or incomplete closure of the eyelids results in corneal dryness, discomfort and possible risk to the cornea

dry macular degeneration see **macular degeneration**

Duane retraction syndrome abnormal function of the rectus muscles wherein the eye retracts into the orbit and the upper eyelid drops when the eye is moved in toward the nose

duction movement of an eye by the extraocular muscles; see also **forced duction test**

dye laser see **laser**

dynamic stabilization method of stabilizing toric contact lenses by thinning the upper and lower edges of the lens, which offer the least resistance to the lids during blinking and thus helps to prevent rotation and maintain the orientation of the lens to correct astigmatism in the proper axis; compare **posterior toric, prism ballast** and **truncation**

dyslexia impairment of reading ability not obviously attributable to any defect within the eye

Ee

Eales disease condition predominantly of young adult males characterized by repeated retinal hemorrhage

eccentric fixation state in which an eye fixates upon an object in such a way that the image of the object does not fall on the fovea, most often as compensation for damage in the area of the fovea

ecchymosis general medical term for discoloration from hemorrhage within a tissue

ectopic general medical term describing a dislocated organ, as in an ectopic lens or pupil

ectropion general medical term for the twisting inside-out of a structure, most commonly in ophthalmic usage referring to a condition in which the lid turns outward from the eye, exposing the conjunctiva

edge glare unwanted scattering of light striking the edge of a contact lens or intraocular lens perceived as streaks or other visual disturbances that reduce visual acuity

edger machine used to trim lenses to fit into spectacle frames

effective power see **back vertex power**

electromagnetic spectrum the range of energy waves conducted through the electrical fields present throughout space, from long-wavelength energy like radio waves to short-wavelength energy like cosmic radiation; visible light includes the wavelengths from about 3800 to about 7600 angstroms, recognized as colors from violet to red, respectively

electro-oculography technique for measuring muscle activity of the eye through electrodes placed on the test subject's face (abbreviation: EOG); changes in electrical potential as the subject alternates the eyes from one fixation point to another are recorded on a strip of paper that runs through the EOG machine

electroretinography technique for measuring the response of the retina to light through electrodes placed on the surface of the globe (abbreviation: ERG)

elevator muscles extraocular muscles that move the eye upward: the superior rectus and inferior oblique

Elschnig bodies or **pearls** small whitish nodules of lens epithelial cells that sometimes appear on remnants of lens capsule after cataract extraction

emmetrope one who does not need corrective lenses to see well at near and far

emmetropia condition in which the unaided eye properly focuses light onto the retina; compare **ametropia**

encircling band elastic band placed around the globe as part of a procedure to repair a retinal detachment

endocapsular appearing or occurring within the lens capsule; see **phacoemulsification**

endolenticular appearing or occurring within the crystalline lens; see **phacoemulsification**

endophthalmitis inflammation of the internal ocular tissues, occasionally an infection after surgery or penetrating injury that can lead to loss of vision and the eye itself if not controlled; **bacterial e.** endophthalmitis caused by infection; **sterile e.** endophthalmitis caused by some agent other than infection

endothelium see **corneal endothelium**

entropion general term for an inward twisting of a structure, most commonly in ophthalmic usage a folding inward of the lid resulting in the lashes rubbing against the globe

enucleation removal of the whole globe of the eye after severing the muscle, nerve and vascular attachments

enucleation implant prosthetic device meant to mimic the appearance of an enucleated eye; see also **orbital implant**

epicanthus fold of facial skin near the inner canthus, especially common and prominent in persons of Asian descent (sometimes called the epicanthal fold)

epikeratophakia refractive surgical procedure in which donor corneal tissue is sutured over the patient's cornea (after removal of the corneal epithelium) to correct myopia, hyperopia or astigmatism

epinucleus tissue surrounding the relatively harder crystalline lens nucleus

epiphora excessive tear flow of the eyes, due either to overproduction of tears or insufficient drainage by the lacrimal system

epiretinal membrane detachment of the internal limiting membrane of the retina from the retina and vitreous body, occurring for a variety of reasons (pathology, surgery or trauma) and sometimes progressing to cellophane maculopathy (wrinkling of the membrane) and macular pucker (contraction of the membrane in the area of the macula)

episclera outermost layer of the sclera containing fine connective tissue and blood vessels

epithelial ingrowth undesirable healing of corneal wounds or incisions in which the corneal epithelium invades the internal surfaces of the healing wound

epithelial punctate keratitis see **keratitis**

epithelium see **corneal epithelium**

equator general term for an imaginary line midway between two poles of a sphere; often used to describe the location of points on the eyeball or crystalline lens (for example, equatorial staphyloma or equatorial cataract)

error see **ametropia**

esophoria heterophoria in which one eye turns inward when deprived of the visual stimulus for fusion

esotropia type of strabismus in which one or both eyes turn in toward the other (also called convergent strabismus); **accommodative e.** esotropia usually appearing in the first few years of life in which excessive turning inward of the eye occurs during near vision; **A-pattern e.** esotropia in which the eyes turn toward each other when the gaze is directed upward; **infantile e.** large esotropia occurring in the first 6 months of life without significant astigmatism or hyperopia; **V-pattern e.** see **A-pattern e.**

ethmoid bone one of the bones of the orbit

ethylenediamine tetra-acetic acid preservative used in some fluid medications; usually given as abbreviation EDTA

eversion general medical term for a turning inside out; in ophthalmic practice, to **evert** the eyelid is to use a cotton swab placed against the outside of the lid to enable the lid to be turned inside out so the palpebral conjunctiva can be examined

evisceration see **enucleation**

evoked potential see **visual evoked potential**

excavation of optic disk see **cupping**

excimer laser see **laser**

executive bifocal classic spectacle design in which the near (reading) segment of the lens extends across the entire width of the bottom of the lens, with a clearly visible line dividing it form the upper far (distance) segment

exenteration see **enucleation**

exfoliation general term for process in which tissue flakes apart in scale-like pieces; in ophthalmic usage, usually describing exfoliation syndrome, the disease process whereby pigment is shed from the iris; compare **pseudoexfoliation syndrome**

exodeviation see **exotropia**

exophoria heterophoria in which an eye turns outward after removal of the visual stimulus

exophthalmia, -os see **proptosis**

exotropia type of strabismus in which one eye is turned away from the other (also called **divergent strabismus**)

exposure keratitis see **keratitis**

expulsive hemorrhage sudden, heavy bleeding from the choroid and retina of the eye, most often occurring during a surgical procedure and having the potential to force ocular tissues out of the incision; it is the most dramatic and potentially most devastating intraoperative complication of ophthalmic surgery

extended wear lens contact lens intended to be worn overnight or, in some cases, up to several weeks without removal; the cornea beneath the lens is able to receive oxygen that is carried in the tear fluid and transmitted through the lens material itself

external limiting membrane of retina layer of the retina in direct contact with the bacillary layer, forming the border with the outer nuclear layer

external rectus muscle see **lateral rectus muscle**

extort to induce motion of an eye so that the "north pole" of the globe tilts outward away from the other eye; compare **intort**

extracapsular cataract extraction general term for surgical techniques in which the anterior lens capsule is partially or completely removed in order to facilitate cataract extraction, usually referring to procedures in which a lens loop is used to remove the lens as an intact unit; see also **capsulorrhexis, capsulotomy, cataract extraction, intracapsular cataract extraction** and **phacoemulsification**

extraocular muscles rectus and oblique muscles attached to the outside of the eye and the inside of the bony orbit, responsible for movements of the eyeball

exudate see **retinal exudates**

exudative retinitis see **retinitis**

eye bank organization that serves as clearing house for donated eyes, most importantly to provide corneas for penetrating keratoplasty but also to distribute eyes unsuitable for transplantation for use in research and training

eyebrow see **supercilium**

eyelash see **cilium**

eyelid either of two flaps of skin that cover the eye during blinking; see also combining forms beginning with *blepharo-*, *palpebro-* and *tarso-*

eye strain see **asthenopia**

Ff

facultative hyperopia see **hyperopia**

facultative suppression mental "blocking out" of image from the deviating eye to prevent it from causing a double image with that of the fixating eye

falciform fold fold of connective tissue where extraocular muscles attach to the globe

Farnsworth test any one of several tests of color vision

far point of accommodation see **accommodation**

far point of convergence see **convergence**

farsightedness see **hyperopia**

fascia general medical term for sheet of fibrous tissue covering an anatomic structure and providing it with attachment, support and protection during movement

fascia bulbi see **Tenon's capsule**

FDA grid collection of data from clinical studies of Food and Drug Administration approved intraocular lenses compiled in the 1980s for use by the FDA in evaluating future trials of IOLs; it includes rates of sight-threatening complications for evaluating safety and postoperative visual acuity data for evaluating effectiveness

fenestrated contact lens see **contact lens**

field see **visual field** and **confrontation field test**

field defect see **visual field defect**

field of view the area in which one can see without turning the head or eyes

filamentary keratitis see **keratitis**

filariasis parasitic infestation with filaria worms, possibly affecting the eyes; see also **onchocerciasis**

filtering bleb see **bleb** and **filtering operation**

filtering operation surgical procedure used in treatment of glaucoma in which an opening is created through which aqueous fluid may pass from the anterior chamber into a sac created beneath the conjunctiva, thus lowering the pressure within the eye

filtration angle see **angle**

finger counting vision see **count-finger vision**

fingerprint corneal dystrophy see **corneal dystrophy**

fish-mouth undesirable postoperative condition in which the edges of a wound or incision fail to close but instead curl and gape open

fixation turning of the eyes toward an object so that the image is placed on the macula, also known as **central f.**; **binocular** or **bifoveal f.** coordination of ocular muscles to bring both eyes to bear upon the same object and bring its image onto the fovea

fixation light or **target** device to assist patient in maintaining fixation during an examination or treatment

flare presence of protein particles in the aqueous humor indicating intraocular inflammation, usually after surgery or trauma; see also **cell**

flare and cell in ophthalmic usage, usually the appearance of white blood cells in the anterior chamber accompanied by the presence of protein particles in the aqueous humor, indicating intraocular inflammation, usually after surgery or trauma

flat in ophthalmic usage, describing the surface curvature of a lens or ocular medium that imparts relatively little refractive power; compare **steep**

flat axis in a toric lens or spherocylindrical ocular medium, the axis of the cylinder

flat chamber collapse of the anterior chamber as a result of insufficient intraocular pressure, typically because of loss of aqueous humor due to trauma or surgical complication

flat top spectacles bifocal spectacles in which the upper half of the lenses impart no refractive power (are plano), prescribed when the wearer needs no distance correction

Fleischer ring a brownish, iron-deposit ring in the corneal epithelium visible on slit lamp examination of eyes with keratoconus

flicker fusion test measure of retinal function in which the frequency of a flashing light is increased until the retinal response "fuses" the flashes into a continuous response

Flieringa ring metal ring placed on the sclera during ophthalmic surgery to maintain the shape of the eye and prevent loss of vitreous humor

floaters dark specks or lines in the field of view caused by cells or other nontransparent material in the vitreous fluid

fluence in optics, the rate of delivery of light energy over time, usually used to described the amount of laser energy being delivered to a treatment area

fluid-gas exchange surgical procedure in which infusion fluid introduced into the posterior chamber as part of retinal detachment repair is removed and replaced by air, a heavy synthetic gas or a mixture of the two

fluorescein yellowish fluorescent dye used in many ophthalmic diagnostic procedures, such as examination of the cornea for lesions or ulcers

fluorescein angiography imaging technique in which fluorescein dye is injected into the arterial system to reveal the circulatory system of the retina and choroid

fluorescein clearance test assessment of the lacrimal system by applying fluorescein drops to the eye and timing how long it takes to drain away with the tear fluid

fluorescein stain topical application of fluorescein to assess the condition of the cornea, especially in evaluation of inflammation and infections

fluorophotometry method for assessing fluid flow (for example, the flow of aqueous humor through the anterior chamber) by measuring the concentration of fluorescein over time using a slit lamp fluorometer

focal distance or **length** distance from a lens to the point at which rays of light converge; if the focal power of a lens in diopters (D) is known, focal length in meters (F) is calculated using the formula $F = 1/D$

focus 1. to bring together rays of light with an optical system so as to obtain an image of an object; 2. the point at which the rays of light converge

fogging technique for eliminating the action of accommodation so that the examiner can determine the amount of astigmatism present; a plus lens is placed before the eye, creating a condition in which accommodation will only further blur the unfocused image, thereby relaxing the accommodation reflex

foldable intraocular lens see **intraocular lens**

follicles in ophthalmic usage, tiny clear or yellow sacs of lymphocytes and inflammatory cells appearing on the conjunctiva after prolonged irritation, often as a result of viral infection

follicular conjunctivitis see **conjunctivitis**

foot-candle measure of the intensity of light falling on a given surface area, defined as one lumen per square foot

foot-lambert another term for foot-candle

forced duction test in ophthalmic usage, intraoperative test of muscle and connective tissue function in which an anesthetized eye is physically moved by the examiner; the ease with which the eye can be moved and the speed with which it returns to a neutral position are observed (also called **passive forced duction test**)

foreign body object lodged in ocular tissue, usually as a result of trauma

foreign body sensation perception that an object is lodged in ocular tissue, either because such an object (sometimes a postoperative suture) is actually present or because of an abrasion, inflammation, trichiasis or other condition

fornix general medical term for an arch-like anatomic structure; in ophthalmic usage, the cul-de-sac (area where the bulbar conjunctiva folds over to become the palpebral conjunctiva)

fovea small pit-like area of the retina in the center of the macula in which cone cells are densely packed, more properly called the fovea centralis; objects must be focused on the fovea in order to be seen in their greatest detail

Fresnel lens (pronounced fray-nell) lens composed of concentric rings that are sections of simple lenses of varying refractive power; used commonly in spotlights because of its ability to remain thin in cross section while providing great focusing power

frontal bone one of the bones of the orbit

front vertex power portion of the total refractive power imparted by the front surface of a lens; compare **back vertex power**

Fuchs dystrophy see **bullous keratopathy** under **keratopathy**

fundus general term for the base of an organ or area (from the Latin for foundation); in ophthalmic usage, the retina and choroid, especially as it appears to an examiner looking in from the front of the eye

funduscopy in ophthalmic usage, viewing the retinal fundus

fusion process by which the brain constructs a single three-dimensional image from the two images transmitted by the eyes; **binocular f.** the production of a single image in the brain from the images on each retina; **motor f.** action of the brain through the oculomotor system to align the eyes to achieve sensory fusion; **sensory f.** action of the brain in combining the images from each eye into one perceived image

fusion amplitude range between the maximum convergence and maximum divergence that a test subject can attain while maintaining fusion at a given level of accommodation; measured by placing base-in and base-out prisms in front of the eyes and adding the power of the maximum prism of each type that can be tolerated before fusion is lost

fusion cards test targets for evaluating fusion or for use in vision training

Gg

Galilean telescope see **telescope**

gamma angle see **angle**

ganglion cell layer retinal cell layer consisting of sensory cells whose axons form the fibers of the optic nerve

gas-fluid exchange surgical procedure in which fluid introduced into the posterior chamber as part of retinal detachment repair is removed and replaced by air, a heavy synthetic gas or a mixture of the two

gas-permeable contact lens see **contact lens**

geniculate body area of the human brain that bridges the optic nerve and the cerebral cortex

giant papillary conjunctivitis see **conjunctivitis**

giant retinal break or **tear** retinal tear extending across three or more clock hours (90°) of the eye

glabella point immediately above the bridge of the nose between the eyebrows, used as a reference point, particularly in reconstructive and plastic surgery

glare distortion in an optical system whereby light from point sources (for example, the sun or automobile headlights) is dispersed across the field of view; glare has been cited as a particular problem for cataract patients, and tests of contrast sensitivity have been proposed as true measures of the visual impairment caused by cataract

glaucoma damage to the optic nerve associated with excessive intraocular pressure, although the pressure level at which damage occurs is completely idiosyncratic and pressure is not the only physiologic mechanism known to be involved in glaucoma; a leading cause of blindness throughout the world, glaucoma in its early stages has no symptoms and causes irreversible vision loss; **acute angle-closure g.** sudden rise in intraocular pressure caused by blockage of the angle of the anterior chamber, marked by painful onset and extremely high pressure; **angle-closure g.** see **closed-angle g.**; **angle-recession g.** high intraocular pressure following blunt trauma to the eye that causes injury to the angle of the anterior chamber with diminished outflow of aqueous fluid; **chronic g.** high intraocular pressure that is sustained over a prolonged time without any critical sudden rises, may be of closed- or open-angle type; **closed-angle g.** glaucoma caused by build-up of aqueous fluid in an anterior chamber that is extremely shallow and thus mechanically prevents normal drainage through the angle; **hemolytic g.** glaucoma caused by blockage of the angle of the anterior chamber by blood cells released by hemorrhage; **iris-block g.** glaucoma caused by adhesions of the iris blocking the normal flow of aqueous humor; **juvenile g.** glaucoma occurring in youth; **low-tension g.** glaucoma occurring at an intraocular pressure usually considered to be within the normal or low range; **malignant g.** elevation of intraocular pressure that continues despite surgical intervention; **neovascular g.** glaucoma caused by growth of blood vessels into the angle of the anterior chamber, which impairs outflow of aqueous fluid; **open-angle g.** glaucoma caused by build-up of aqueous fluid in the anterior chamber, even though the angle is open, due to impaired outflow through the tissue spaces of the angle; **phacolytic g.** glaucoma resulting from leakage of lens proteins in very advanced cases of cataract; **pigmentary** or **pigmentary dispersion g.** glaucoma resulting from iris pigment dispersed into the anterior chamber; **primary g.** general term for glaucoma resulting from no previous disease (generally divided into primary closed-angle and primary open-angle glaucoma); **pupillary block g.** glaucoma caused by build-up of aqueous fluid behind the iris, which is adherent to the crystalline lens and traps aqueous; **secondary g.** glaucoma resulting from disease or injury (compare **primary g.**)

glaucomatous like or of glaucoma

glaucomatous cataract opacification caused by high intraocular pressure

glaucomatous cupping see **cupping**

globe another term for the eyeball

goblet cells mucin-producing cells found in mucous membranes; in the eye, goblet cells are located in the conjunctiva and produce the mucin found in tears

Goldmann applanation tonometer see **tonometer**

Goldmann lens see **goniolens**

Goldmann tonometer see **tonometer**

goniolens lens, typically incorporating several mirrors, that allows one to see or direct laser energy into the angle of the anterior chamber when it is placed onto the anesthetized eye; many configurations are available, including the Goldmann, Hruby, Karickhoff and Zeiss lenses

goniophotocoagulation laser procedure for treatment of glaucoma that attempts to control intraocular pressure by using laser energy to destroy aqueous-producing tissues in the angle

gonioscopy examination of the angle of the anterior chamber using a goniolens

grade I, II, III and **IV** many medical conditions, including ophthalmic entities such as capsular opacification, cataract, corneal haze, etc., are assessed by assigning grades from I (or 1, noticeable) to IV (or 4, severe); although some researchers periodically attempt to define objective criteria for the grades assigned to these various conditions, virtually none of these attempts at standardization make any impression upon clinicians (who prefer to establish their own definitions for use in patient records)

Graefe knife surgical instrument once widely used in cataract extraction, now largely abandoned

grid see **Amsler grid** or **FDA grid**

Gunn pupil see **Marcus Gunn pupil**

guttata general medical colloquialism for a spot or spots with the appearance of water droplets, in ophthalmic usage referring to the appearance of such spots on the inner surface of the cornea (see **endothelial corneal dystrophy** under **corneal dystrophy**); plural: indeterminable; the English term guttata seems to be a derivative of Latin-named conditions such as cornea guttata, which actually translates to guttate cornea; however, most speakers and writers erroneously transform the Latin phrase into English as corneal guttata, then use **guttata** to describe the entity correctly called a gutta (the correct Latin plural of which is guttae); even though the term guttata is found in authoritative medical dictionaries only as an adjective as described above, its misapplication to describe a droplet-like corneal spot is so well established in common ophthalmic usage that spurious plurals such as guttatae and guttatas have now proliferated in the literature, as has the usage of guttata as a singular nominative case noun; no matter how hard this author tried, he could come to no reasonable decision on a correct singular or plural form (you might as well go ahead and use guttata as the singular and guttatae as the plural—they seem to be well accepted)

Hh

half-glasses spectacles that have only the lower half of a lens, used to provide correction for near vision to presbyopes who find their uncorrected distance vision acceptable

halo distortion in an optical system that causes rings of light to be seen around point sources of light

hand-motion vision very low level of visual acuity in which no greater detail can be perceived than the motion of a hand waved before the eyes; see also **count-finger vision, light perception vision, no light perception vision** and **visual acuity**

haploscope instrument that presents two separate fields of view to the two eyes for evaluation of binocular vision

haptic portion of an intraocular lens comprising a thin arm that curves outward from the optic, sometimes referred to as a "loop"

hard exudates see **retinal exudates**

harmonious retinal correspondence state in which corresponding points from the two images focused on each retina are properly associated in the image created by fusion in the brain; compare **anomalous retinal correspondence**

haze general term in ophthalmic usage for cloudiness of normally clear optical medium, usually referring to the cornea

heavy fluid or **gas** any of several materials used in posterior segment surgery to replace the vitreous humor following vitrectomy, often as part of retinal detachment repair; these materials include perfluorocarbons such as perfluoropropane (C_3F_8), silicone oil, sulfur hexafluoride (SF_6)

hemianopia, -opsia partial or total loss of vision in half the visual field, resulting from some extraocular defect so that the visual field of both eyes can be affected; the upper or lower portions of the visual field, as well as the nasal and temporal sides, can be affected; **absolute h.** total loss of all visual perception in half the visual field; **bilateral** or **binocular h.** partial or total loss of vision affecting the visual field of both eyes (also called *true hemianopia*); **nasal h.** loss of the half of the visual field on the side nearest the nose; **quadrantic h.** loss of one quarter of the visual field; **relative h.** loss of certain visual perceptions (for example, color) in half the visual field; **temporal h.** loss of the half of the visual field on the side nearest the temple; **unilateral h.** loss of half the visual field of only one eye

hemiopia loss of light perception across half the retina

HeNe laser see **laser**

Henle's fibers nerve fibers that join the rod and cone cells of the retina in the area of the fovea

Hering's law of simultaneous innervation physiologic principle that the nerve stimulus generate by the oculomotor system to move the fixating eye is duplicated for the yoke muscle of the other eye, resulting in parallel movement of the eyes

herpes zoster ophthalmicus viral infection affecting the trigeminal nerve and the eye

heterochromic general anatomic term describing a tissue or organ that shows a mottling of colors when normally it is a single hue (for example, a heterochromic iris)

heteronymous diplopia double vision in which the image seen by the right eye is perceived to be to the left of the image seen by the left eye (also known as **crossed diplopia**)

heteronymous field defect visual field defect in which the halves of each field (for example, both left halves of each visual field) are not the same

heterophoria failure of fusion in which one or both eyes involuntarily deviate from their fixation axes when the object of fixation is suddenly removed; see also **anisophoria, cataphoria, hyperphoria** and **hypophoria**; compare **orthophoria**

heterophthalmia general term for difference in structure or function between the two eyes

heteropsia state in which one eye has different visual characteristics (for example, degree of myopia) than the fellow eye

heterotropia see **strabismus**

hippus rhythmic contraction and dilation of the pupils independent of any stimulus, often seen when shining a light into the eye in order to evaluate pupillary reflexes; not usually indicative of pathology

Hirschberg test measurement of tropia by noting the position of the reflections on the corneas of the test subject of a fixation light held by the examiner; if both reflections are centered on the pupils, the eyes are orthotropic, but if the reflection is centered on one pupil but not the other, a tropia may be present

homonymous diplopia double vision in which the image seen by the right eye is perceived to be to the right of the image seen by the left eye (also known as *uncrossed diplopia*)

homonymous field defect visual field defect in which the halves of each field (for example, both left halves of each visual field) are the same

Honan balloon device placed on the eye before ophthalmic surgery; its pressure upon the eye eventually causes a reduction in intraocular pressure

hordeolum infection of one of the glands on the edge of the eyelid (**external h.**) or in the palpebral conjunctiva (**internal h.**); see also **chalazion** and **meibomian cyst**

horizontal prism bar see **prism bar**

horopter general term for method of correlating points in space to points on the retina for given conditions of fixation, binocularity, etc.

horseshoe tear retinal tear in which a flap of retinal tissue attached on one side is pulled away from the retina by its attachment to the vitreous body

HOTV test visual acuity test for children in which the letters H, O, T and V on a chart are matched to the same letters on cards

Hruby contact lens see **goniolens**

humor general term for a fluid; **aqueous h.** see **aqueous; vitreous h.** see **vitreous body**

hyaloid membrane in ophthalmic usage, the thin membrane that surrounds the vitreous, consists of anterior hyaloid membrane (also called the vitreous face) and posterior hyaloid membrane

hyaluronic acid component of certain viscoelastic substances

hydrodelamination or **hydrodelineation** in ophthalmic usage, surgical technique in which fluid is injected into the lens nucleus in order to break it up in order to facilitate cataract extraction

hydrodissection most often in ophthalmic usage, surgical technique in which water is injected between tissue layers in order to separate them, usually employed in cataract extraction to separate the lens nucleus from the surrounding cortex; see also **viscodissection**

hydrogel material used to make contact lenses and intraocular lenses; the hydrogel polymer (centered around the HEMA or hydroxyethylmethacrylate molecule) is hydrophilic, which means that it can absorb large amounts of water and theoretically is more friendly living tissue than hydrophobic materials

hydrophilic describing a material that mixes with water

hydrophobic describing a material that repels water

hydrops general medical term for accumulation of watery fluid in tissue; **corneal h.** accumulation of aqueous fluid within the cornea as a result of the loss of tissue integrity of the corneal endothelium and Descemet's membrane

hydroxyethylmethacrylate see **hydrogel**

hypermature cataract see **cataract**

hypermetropia see **hyperopia**

hyperope individual with hyperopia

hyperopia visual defect in which the eye focuses rays of light so that the focal point is behind the retina; commonly known as farsightedness, the hyperopic eye is not able to see objects that are nearby; **axial h.** farsightedness attributable to the length of the eye, that is, the eye is too short for the refractive power of the cornea and crystalline lens; **facultative h.** amount of farsightedness inherent in the refractive system of the eye that is normally compensated for by accommodation; **refractive h.** farsightedness that is attributable to the refractive power of the eye, that is, the cornea and lens are too weak to bring the incoming rays of light to focus on the retina

hyperopic keratomileusis or **LASIK** see **keratomileusis**

hyperphoria heterophoria in which the eyes move upward after removal of the visual stimulus

hypertelorism general medical term for abnormally large distance between two anatomic structures; in ophthalmic usage, an abnormally large distance between the eyes, a congenital condition usually accompanied by problems with ocular alignment and motility

hypertropia strabismus in which the non-fixating eye points upward relative to the fixating eye

hyphema bleeding into the anterior chamber of the eye

hypophoria heterophoria in which the eyes move downward after removal of the visual stimulus

hypopyon collection of pus in the anterior chamber of the eye

hypotelorism general medical term for abnormally small distance between two anatomic structures; in ophthalmic usage, an abnormally small distance between the eyes

hypotony in ophthalmic usage, low intraocular pressure

hypotropia strabismus in which the non-fixating eye points downward relative to the fixating eye

hysterical blindness see **blindness**

Ii

illiterate E vision test target used for subjects who cannot read; the letter E is arranged in different directions and different sizes, and the subject indicates which direction the "fork" of the letter E is pointing

implant general term for man-made material designed for surgical insertion into the human body; see also **intraocular lens** and **enucleation implant**

incident light ray of light that strikes a surface and is absorbed, reflected and/or refracted; see also **reflection** and **refraction**

inclusion bodies or **inclusions** general medical term for foreign particles seen in cells or tissues where they do not belong, in ophthalmic usage often referring to particles of an unknown nature seen in the cornea

inclusion conjunctivitis see **conjunctivitis**

incomitant adjective describing a varying relationship between the lines of sight of the two eyes that depends upon the direction of gaze, usually a result of an extraocular muscle problem; compare **concomitant**

incomitant strabismus see **strabismus**

incongruous general term indicating dissimilarity in form

incongruous field defect the presence of visual field defects in both eyes that do not match each other

incongruous hemianopia loss of half the visual field in each eye, but with a dissimilarity of the size and/or shape of the defect in each eye

index of refraction see **refractive index**

indirect illumination in slit lamp biomicroscopy, method of viewing an ocular structure by reflected light in which the slit lamp light source is shined upon some other ocular structure than the one to be viewed; see also **retroillumination,** compare **direct illumination**

indirect lens a hand-held lens system used during indirect ophthalmoscopy

indirect ophthalmoscopy process of viewing the internal structures of the eye through instrumentation, usually consisting of a light source and lens/prism viewer worn on the examiner's head and a hand-held lens placed on the cornea, that presents the upside-down, reversed image of the interior of the eye; the examiner uses both eyes to view the subject, thus obtaining a three-dimensional image; compare **direct ophthalmoscopy**

induced in ophthalmic surgical usage, usually referring to a condition that is a result (often unwanted) of surgery, such as induced astigmatism following cataract surgery; see also **consecutive**

infantile general medical term describing a feature or process (for example, glaucoma or cataract) that occurs in early childhood; compare **senile**

inferior oblique muscle extraocular muscle lying underneath the eye around the equator of the globe responsible for elevating, abducting and extorting the eye

inferior rectus muscle extraocular muscle lying underneath the eye responsible for adducting, depressing and extorting the eye

infiltrates small particles that appear in tissue that is normally free of such particles; **corneal i.** whitish, cloudy particles in the cornea, often associated with infection or contact lens wear; **sterile i.** infiltrates, usually of the cornea, that are not associated with infection

infiltrative keratitis see **keratitis**

infinity in optics, imaginary point at great distance from which rays of light travel in parallel paths; in clinical settings, 20 feet or more is considered to be infinity (thus the denominator 20 for distance acuity measured using the Snellen test chart)

infraorbital at the bottom of or beneath the bony eye socket

infusion the act of introducing fluid into a closed anatomic structure, usually during surgery, or the fluid itself; see also **irrigation**

injection 1. the act of introducing fluid into tissue through a needle; 2. condition in which tissue is red, swollen and engorged with dilated blood vessels, most often in ophthalmic usage referring to conjunctival injection

inner granular or **molecular layer of retina** cell layer with in the retina composed primarily of nerve synapses and containing the amacrine cells, located between the ganglion cell layer and the inner nuclear layer; see also **retina**

inner nuclear layer of retina cell layer within the retina composed primarily of bipolar cells and containing the capillaries that supply blood to the retina, located between the inner and outer molecular layers; see also **retina**

insufficiency see **accommodative insufficiency** and **convergence insufficiency**

intermittent not present at all times; see definitions for **intermittent esotropia, intermittent exotropia** and **intermittent strabismus** under main words

internal limiting membrane of the retina innermost layer of the retina, in direct contact with the vitreous humor, also called the hyaloid face of the vitreous; see also **retina**

internal rectus muscle see **medial rectus muscle**

interocular or **interpupillary distance** see **pupillary distance**

intort to induce motion of an eye so that the "north pole" of the globe tilts inward toward the other eye; compare **extort**

intracameral general medical term describing an entity located or occurring within a chamber; in ophthalmic usage either within the anterior or posterior chamber

intracameral anesthesia anesthetic agent injected into the anterior chamber of the eye, usually during cataract surgery

intracapsular cataract extraction general term for surgical techniques in which cataract extraction is accomplished either by grasping with forceps or cryoextraction while the lens remains within its intact capsule (abbreviation: ICCE); ICCE has been almost completely abandoned (except in economically underdeveloped areas of the world) in favor of extracapsular procedures; see also **capsulotomy, cataract extraction, extracapsular cataract extraction** and **phacoemulsification**

intracapsular ligament connective tissue joining the extraocular muscles to the globe

intracorneal within the cornea

intracorneal implant see **intrastromal corneal ring**

intraocular general anatomic term for structure or process appearing or occurring within the eye

intraocular lens artificial lens surgically implanted into the eye to correct a refractive error, especially after cataract extraction (abbreviation: IOL); the age of contemporary intraocular lenses is considered to have begun in 1949 with the first implantation of an IOL made of polymethylmethacrylate; contemporary IOLs are manufactured in many designs from a variety of materials, but all have in common a central focusing portion (the optic) and a supporting structure (the haptics); **acrylic IOL** foldable IOL manufactured from a polymer containing acrylic materials; **anterior chamber IOL** or **lens (ACL)** IOL designed to be implanted in front of the iris, either after cataract extraction to correct aphakia or with the crystalline lens still in place to correct a refractive error (compare **posterior chamber IOL**); **C-loop IOL** IOL whose haptics are shaped like the letter C; **disk IOL** IOL with one circular haptic, designed to be implanted in the lens capsule to achieve centration; **foldable IOL** lens implant that can be folded, by virtue of either lens design or choice of soft lens material, and inserted into the eye through a small incision; **hydrogel IOL** foldable IOL manufactured from a polymer based upon the hydroxyethyl-methacrylate (HEMA) molecule; **J-loop IOL** IOL whose haptics are shaped like the letter J; **piggyback IOLs** implantation of two IOLs in the same eye in order to achieve higher refractive power than possible with a single IOL; **plate-haptic IOL** IOL designed with flat, more or less solid plates instead of "arms" for haptics; **posterior chamber IOL** or **lens (PCL)** IOL designed to be implanted behind the iris, in either the lens capsule ("in the bag") or in the ciliary sulcus (compare **anterior chamber IOL**); **secondary IOL** IOL implanted in a separate procedure some time after the crystalline lens has been removed, usually because some intraoperative complication prevented IOL implantation at the time of the first procedure; **silicone IOL** foldable IOL manufactured from a polymer based upon the silicone molecule; **soft IOL** see **foldable IOL**

intraocular lens exchange surgical procedure to remove one intraocular lens and replace it with another, either to replace a damaged or dislocated IOL or to insert the appropriate power lens if the first lens failed to correct vision sufficiently

intraocular pressure pressure within the eye, measured like atmospheric pressure as the height of a column of mercury that the pressure can support, thus the unit of measure mm Hg (abbreviation: IOP); see also **glaucoma, hypotony** and **ocular hypertension**

intraorbital within the bony eye socket

intraorbital implant device, usually composed of a bone-like substance, implanted in the orbit after the eye is removed due to disease; often designed to accept a prosthetic eye

intrastromal general medical term for location within the main substance of a tissue; in ophthalmic usage referring to the corneal stroma

intrastromal corneal ring device, shaped like a lens, ring or portion of a ring, implanted within the cornea to correct a refractive error

intravitreal located with the vitreous humor

intumescent cataract see **cataract**

irid- root word meaning iris

iridectomy surgical procedure to remove iris tissue; **peripheral i.** removal of a small piece of iris tissue near its edge (away from the pupil) to facilitate the flow of aqueous humor and thus lower or prevent a rise in intraocular pressure;

sector i. iridectomy in which a portion of the iris from the edge of the pupil to the outer edge of the iris is removed (resulting in a keyhole pupil); **total i.** see **sector i.;** compare **iridotomy**

iridemia bleeding from the iris

irides plural of iris

iridocorneal angle see **angle**

iridocorneal endothelial syndrome condition in which corneal and iris endothelial cells proliferate, causing adhesions between the iris and cornea as well as blocking the iridocorneal angle, resulting in intraocular pressure rise

iridocyclitis inflammation of the iris and ciliary body

iridodialysis detachment of the root of the iris from the ciliary body

iridodonesis abnormal anteroposterior movement ("flopping") of the iris

iridoplegia partial or total paralysis of the iris

iridotomy surgical procedure to create an opening in the iris; see also **laser iridotomy;** compare **iridectomy**

iris mobile, vascular, ring-shaped structure whose movements control the size of the pupil, and thus the amount of light passing through to the retina, attached at its outer edge to the ciliary body and covered with a (usually) highly pigmented epithelial layer (plural: irides); the pupillary zone of the iris contains the iris sphincter (sphincter pupillae), which constricts the pupil, and the ciliary zone contains the outer dilator muscle (dilator pupillae), which dilates the pupil; between them lies the colarette; the iris is usually considered the division between the anterior and posterior chambers of the eye, although surgical procedures involving the lens and ciliary body, both of which lie behind the iris, are described as anterior segment surgery

iris-block glaucoma see **glaucoma**

iris bombé "ballooning" of the iris outward into the anterior chamber caused by a build-up of fluid behind the iris; see also **pupillary block**

iris coloboma see **coloboma**

iris crypts normally occurring furrows in the front surface of the iris

iris hooks surgical instruments used to catch the edge of the iris and pull and hold open the pupil to facilitate surgery

iris nevus small area, either smooth or slightly elevated, of excess pigment on the iris

iris prolapse protrusion of part of the iris through a wound or surgical incision

iris root area of the iris where it inserts into the ciliary body

iris sphincter circular muscle within the iris surrounding the pupil and responsible for constriction of the pupil

iritis inflammation of the iris

iron lines brown to black lines in the cornea caused by iron deposits

irregular astigmatism see **astigmatism**

irrigation general surgical term for introduction of fluid to an area

irrigation and aspiration surgical instrument and technique for removing intraocular tissue by simultaneously injecting fluid (irrigation) and applying suction (aspiration); abbreviation: I&A or I/A; several different instruments have been specially designed to perform irrigation and aspiration for various ophthalmic applications

ischemic optic neuropathy injury to the optic nerve because of a loss of blood flow, usually resulting in sudden blindness

iseikonia normal condition in which each eye receives an image of similar size; compare **aniseikonia**

Ishihara test test for color vision

isochromatic uniformity of color, either between two or more objects (as in some vision test targets for color blindness) or between different parts of the same object (as in an iris that is of a uniform color); compare **anisochromatic**

isocoria normal condition in which the pupils of the two eyes are the same size; compare **anisocoria**

isometropia state in which both eyes have the same refractive power; compare **anisometropia**

isopter general term for line on a chart or map connecting similar numerical values; in ophthalmic usage, lines on a visual field test chart connecting similar test results

Jj

Jackson cross cylinder lens see **cross cylinder**

Jaeger acuity measurement of visual acuity at near distances (reading acuity) based upon standard sizes of printed block letters, recorded as J1, J2, etc.; see also **Snellen acuity**

J-loop lens see **intraocular lens**

juvenile describing a feature or process (for example, cataract or glaucoma) appearing or occurring in late childhood; compare **infantile**

Kk

kappa angle see **angle**

Karickhoff lens see **goniolens**

Kelman phacoemulsification see **phaco-emulsification**

kerat-, -o- root word meaning literally *horn,* usually referring to the cornea but also describing other "hard" tissues such as fingernails

keratectomy general term for surgical removal of corneal tissue, usually performed as part of a corneal graft procedure (see **keratoplasty**); also, excimer laser surgery is described as photorefractive keratectomy because wide areas of corneal tissue are removed

keratic precipitates small white or yellow bodies composed of inflammatory cells that adhere to the corneal endothelium, usually in the lower portion of the anterior chamber, seen in cases of iritis and iridocyclitis; **granulomatous** or **mutton-fat k.p.** large keratic precipitates resulting from long-standing inflammatory conditions; **punctate k.p.** small keratic precipitates

keratitis general term for inflammation of the cornea; *Acanthamoeba* k. inflammation of the cornea resulting from an infection with the **Acanthamoeba** organism, almost always associated with contact lens wear; **annular k.** inflammation and appearance of deposits around the periphery of the cornea; **band k.** see

keratopathy; dendriform or **dendritic k.** branched lesion appearing on the cornea in herpes virus infections; **disciform k.** appearance of round opacity deep in corneal tissue, usually chronic but not dangerous, often as a result of previous viral infection or trauma; **epithelial punctate k.** see **superficial punctate k.; exposure k.** condition of corneal dryness, usually resulting from deficiency of tear fluid and/or incomplete closure of the eyelids during sleep; **filamentary k.** appearance of filaments attached to the corneal epithelium, can be a result of many conditions such as dry eye, infection, corneal abrasion, etc.; **herpes** or **herpetic k.** herpes virus infection leading to inflammation and appearance of lesions that may progress to ulcers on the cornea; **infiltrative k.** corneal inflammation associated with whitish, cloudy particles, often indicating an infection or sometimes as a result of contact lens wear; **lattice k.** see **lattice corneal dystrophy; punctate k.** condition in which precipitates form in small points on the corneal endothelium; **superficial punctate k.** condition in which precipitates form in small points on the corneal epithelium

keratitis sicca see **keratoconjunctivitis sicca**

keratoconjunctivitis inflammation of the tissues of the cornea and conjunctiva simultaneously; **atopic k.** keratoconjunctivitis associated with unusual sensitivity to allergens; **phlyctenular k.** inflammation of the cornea and conjunctiva associated with the appearance of small blisters

on the cornea and conjunctiva; see also
phlyctenule

keratoconjunctivitis sicca condition in which
there is dryness, redness and itching of the
cornea and conjunctiva, often associated with
chronic insufficient tear production; see also
dry eye syndrome

keratoconus malformation of the cornea such that
it is thin and cone-like in shape rather than
rounded

keratoglobus malformation of the cornea such
that it is thin and protrudes in a globe-like
shape

keratomalacia progressive degeneration of the
cornea as a result of vitamin A deficiency

keratome surgical instrument used to cut the
cornea, either to create an incision into the eye
for cataract surgery or to slice across the cornea
to create a button for transplantation or flap for
refractive surgery; see also **keratoplasty** and
microkeratome

keratometer any of several types of instrument
used to measure the curvature of the cornea;
see also **corneal topography**

keratometry general term for measurement of the
cornea, either of corneal thickness (see
pachymetry) or of corneal curvature (see
keratoscopy)

keratomileusis any of several refractive surgical procedures in which a keratome is used to remove and/or reshape corneal tissue to correct a refractive error; **automated lamellar k.** see entry under **keratoplasty; Barraquer k.** procedure no longer in use in which corneal tissue was removed, frozen, reshaped, thawed and replaced on the eye; **hyperopic k.** keratomileusis performed to correct farsightedness; **laser in situ k.** keratomileusis in which a keratome is used to remove an outer layer of corneal tissue, a laser is used to reshape the exposed corneal tissue and then the outer layer of corneal tissue is replaced (this technique is usually written and spoken as its abbreviation: LASIK); **myopic k.** keratomileusis performed to correct nearsightedness

keratopathy general term for unhealthy condition of the cornea; **band k.** condition, usually resulting from some underlying ocular or systemic disease, marked by calcium deposits in Bowman's layer which, as the name implies, appear across the cornea in narrow bands; **bullous k.** degenerative condition of the cornea in which the epithelial cells form small blisters (bullae) that eventually burst; usually the result of some previous ocular disease; **pseudophakic bullous k.** degenerative condition of the cornea resulting from improper intraocular lens implantation in which the endothelial cells form bullae; **ribbon k.** see **band k.;** see also **keratitis**

keratophakia refractive surgical procedure in which a thin slice of cornea is removed, then replaced over a suitably shaped piece of donor cornea (called a lenticle)

keratoplasty general term for corneal grafting procedures, in which a patient's cornea is removed with a keratome and replaced with donor tissue (as is commonly done in cases of corneal disease) or (as is done in some refractive surgical procedures) after being reshaped; **automated lamellar k.** procedure in which a keratome is used first to remove an outer layer of corneal tissue and then to remove an inner layer of tissue; the outer layer of tissue is then replaced on the eye, with the shape of the removed inner layer determining the change in the refractive state of the eye; **lamellar k.** surgical procedure to treat corneal opacity by removing a layer of corneal tissue in the area of the opacity and replacing it with a clear corneal graft; **penetrating k.** surgical procedure to treat corneal opacity in which the entire depth of a section of cornea is removed and replaced by a graft (colloquially known as corneal transplantation); **refractive k.** general term for keratoplasty performed to correct a refractive error rather than an opacity

keratoprosthesis artificial device used to replace the cornea either permanently in an attempt to restore sight (rarely used and rarely successful) or temporarily to facilitate some other operative procedure prior to replacing the cornea with a graft

keratorefractive surgery see **refractive surgery**

keratoscopy technique for measuring the shape of the cornea by projecting evenly spaced, concentric circles of light (keratometric mires) onto it; irregularities of the shape of the circles or the width of the space between them show deviations from a perfectly spherical shape; see also **Placido disk**

keratotomy surgical procedure in which incisions are made into the cornea; usually referring to refractive surgical procedures in which incisions are carefully placed in the cornea so that the natural healing response and structural changes that ensue will reshape the cornea and correct any refractive errors present; **arcuate** or **astigmatic k.** keratotomy consisting of curved incisions (with the arc centered on the optical axis) performed to correct astigmatism; **delimiting k.** obsolete (and generally ineffective) procedure for limiting the spread of a corneal ulcer by making incisions around it; **radial k.** refractive surgical procedure in which corneal incisions are placed radially, like the spokes of a wheel (leaving a central optical zone free of incisions), in order to flatten the cornea and correct nearsightedness (abbreviation: RK); the degree of flattening depends upon the depth (about 90% of the corneal thickness) and number (typically from four to eight) of incisions

keyhole pupil condition of the eye following a sector iridectomy in which the pupil resembles a keyhole

kinetic perimetry see **perimetry**

Koeppe lens see **goniolens**

K-reading usually the measurement of corneal shape (see **keratoscopy**), but sometimes referring to measurement of corneal thickness (see **pachymetry**)

Krimsky measurement measurement of the angle of tropia by determining how much prism power must be placed in front of the subject's eye to center in the pupils the reflections of a fixation light held by the examiner

Krukenberg's spindles vertical linear deposits of small dots of pigment on the corneal endothelium appearing in uveitis or pigment dispersion syndrome

Krupin implant, shunt or **valve** device implanted to control intraocular pressure by allowing aqueous fluid to flow from the anterior chamber into a filtering bleb

Ll

lacri- root word meaning tears; also see **dacry-**

lacrimal apparatus system that produces tears and allows them to drain from the eye; it includes the lacrimal glands (which produce tear fluid), the puncta (openings inside each upper and lower eyelid through which tear fluid drains from the eye), the lacrimal sac (which holds the overflow of tears), the lacrimal ducts or canaliculi (tubes that lead to the nasolacrimal duct), and the nasolacrimal duct (through which tears then drain into the nasal passages)

lacrimal bone one of the bones of the orbit

lacrimal caruncle small mound of conjunctival tissue in the medial canthus

lacrimal intubation surgical procedure in which tubes are implanted in a blocked lacrimal duct in order to restore tear drainage

lacrimal probing surgical procedure in which a flexible probe is passed through the lacrimal duct in order to clear a blockage

lacrimation flow of tears

lactoferrin protein produced by the lacrimal gland and found in tear fluid

lactoferrin test test in which a filter paper is placed on the eye to absorb tear fluid, then is placed on a reactive plate that indicates the amount of lactoferrin present in the tears; in dry eye syndrome, lactoferrin levels are lower than normal

lagophthalmos incomplete closure of eyelids, which may result in exposure keratitis

lambda angle *see* **angle**

lamellar adjective describing a structure or process occurring in layers; partial-depth corneal transplants (as opposed to penetrating keratoplasty) are often described as lamellar grafts

lamellar keratoplasty *see* **keratoplasty**

lamina cribrosa mesh-like area of sclera at the back of the eye through which retinal ganglion cells and blood vessels pass

Landolt ring vision test chart containing targets in the shape of circles, each with a small section of its circumference removed; the subject must identify the orientation of the breaks

lase to emit coherent light

laser acronym for Light Amplification by Stimulated Emission of Radiation, a process invented in the early 1960s to produce coherent light (that is, light of a single frequency whose waves are in phase); there are many types of lasers with diverse medical applications, all of which are based upon the fact that specific wavelengths of light are absorbed by specific tissues or compounds within tissues, with various consequent reactions; **argon l.** laser in which the light source is argon gas excited by electricity, producing laser energy in the blue-green part of the electromagnetic spectrum, which is absorbed by the red pigments of vascular tissue; current ophthalmic applications include treatment of diabetic retinopathy and macular degeneration, as well as trabeculoplasty and iridotomy; **carbon dioxide (CO_2) l.** laser in which the light source is carbon dioxide gas, producing laser energy at a fundamental wavelength of 10,600 nanometers; ophthalmic applications include removal of tumors from the orbit and cosmetic resurfacing of skin around the eyes; **diode l.** laser in which light is produced by electrical excitation of a solid-state semiconductor; **dye l.** laser in which a source of lased light is directed through a liquid dye that controls the wavelength of the energy that finally exits the laser; **erbium:yttrium-aluminum-garnet (Er:YAG) l.** laser in which an Er:YAG crystal is excited by electricity and induced to emit laser light; ophthalmic applications include cosmetic procedures of the skin around the eyes and removal of cataracts; **excimer l.** laser in which the light source is an electrically excited dimer: a gas with two component elements, such as argon and fluorine; argon fluoride excimer lasers are currently used in ophthalmic practice to reshape the cornea by the process of photoablation; **helium-neon (HeNe) l.** laser producing light of a visible wavelength used as an aiming beam for ophthalmic surgical lasers that operate at wavelengths that are not visible; **mode-locked l.** type of Q-switched laser that employs a dye; **neodymium:yttrium-aluminum-garnet (Nd:YAG) l.** laser in which an Nd:YAG crystal is excited by electricity and induced to emit laser light of infrared wavelength; the principal ophthalmic application of the Nd:YAG laser is posterior capsulotomy, although there are applications in vitreous and glaucoma surgery; **Q-switched l.** general term for lasers that concentrate energy into short pulses by employing filters to prevent light from exiting the laser until a certain threshold of energy is achieved; **ruby l.** original laser using an electric arc to produce light that is made coherent by a rod composed of synthetic ruby crystal; **YAG l.** see **Nd:YAG l.**

laser in situ keratomileusis see **keratomileusis**

laser iridotomy creation of a hole in the peripheral iris using a laser; performed to enhance the flow of aqueous humor and lower intraocular pressure in eyes with glaucoma

laser trabeculoplasty destruction of small areas of the trabecular meshwork using a laser; performed to reduce the production of aqueous humor and lower intraocular pressure in eyes with glaucoma

lateral general anatomic term describing a structure or process appearing or occurring at the side; in ophthalmic usage, referring to the side of the eye nearest the temple; see also **temporal;** compare **medial** and **nasal**

lateral angle see **lateral canthus**

lateral canthus area where the upper and lower eyelids join at the side of the face nearest the temple; also called the temporal canthus and lateral angle; compare **medial canthus**

lateral geniculate body area of the midbrain that receives visual impulses from the nerve fibers of the optic tract

lateral rectus muscle extraocular muscle lying along the side of the eye near the temple and responsible for abducting the eye

lattice degeneration of the retina condition in which the retinal tissues thin and blood vessels harden (leading to the "lattice" appearance), with break-up of the internal limiting membrane and adhesion of the vitreous to the retina; although most eyes with lattice degeneration do not progress to retinal detachment, in eyes with retinal detachments about one-third have lattice degeneration as the underlying cause

lattice dystrophy of the cornea progressive condition, usually beginning around puberty, in which lines of opacification appear through the corneal stroma and slowly increase in thickness and number

lazy eye colloquial term for amblyopia

legal blindness see **blindness**

lens general term for a transparent object that bends light rays from their original path, either to bring them together to a focus or spread them apart; compare **prism;** see also **Bagolini l., biconcave l., biconvex l., bifocal l., bitoric l., concave l., convex l., crystalline l., goniolens, intraocular l., minus l., multifocal l., plus l., slab-off l., spherical l.** and **trial l.**

lens blank unfinished spectacle or contact lens that does not yet exhibit its final refractive power

lens capsule thin, transparent membrane surrounding the crystalline lens to which the zonules are attached

lensectomy surgical procedure in which the crystalline lens is removed

lens epithelium the one-cell-thick layer of epithelial cells that covers the crystalline lens of the eye; when left in the lens capsule after cataract extraction they can proliferate to form Elschnig's pearls

lens glide surgical instrument used to support and guide an intraocular lens as it is being implanted into the eye

lens loop surgical instrument consisting of a handle with a small loop at the end, usually notched with small "teeth," that is used to remove the crystalline lens during extracapsular cataract extraction

lensmeter instrument used to measure the various components of curvature, and thus the refractive properties, of an artificial lens

lens nucleus see **nucleus**

lens vault *s*ee definition 1 under **apical clearance**

lenticle *s*mall "button" of donor corneal ti*s*sue used in refractive keratoplasty; *s*ee al*s*o **keratophakia**

lenticular general term meaning of or like a lens, commonly referring to the natural crystalline lens of the eye

lenticular astigmatism *s*ee **astigmatism**

lenticular cataract opacity of the crystalline len*s*; *s*ee al*s*o **cataract**

lenticule *s*ee **lenticle**

leukoma den*s*e white opacity of the cornea

levator muscle mu*s*cle that lift*s* the upper eyelid

lid either of two flap*s* of *s*kin that cover the eye during blinking; *s*ee al*s*o combining form*s* beginning with blepharo-, palpebro- and tarso-

lid lag delay in downward motion of upper eyelid when the eye look*s* downward; *s*ee al*s*o **von Graefe's sign**

lid retraction opening of upper and/or lower lid wider than normal, re*s*ulting in exce*s*sive exposure of *s*clera

lid speculum in*s*trument u*s*ed to hold the eyelid*s* open

light portion of the electromagnetic *s*pectrum visible to the human eye

light perception vision very low visual acuity in which the subject can perceive only the presence or absence of light and is unable to see objects; see also **count-finger vision, hand-motion vision, no light perception vision** and **visual acuity**

limbal general medical term meaning near the line along which two structures meet; in ophthalmic usage, usually referring to the circular border between the cornea and sclera

limbal conjunctiva see **conjunctiva**

limbus general anatomic term for the line along which two structures meet; most commonly in ophthalmic usage, the circular border between the cornea and sclera

limiting membranes of retina see **retina**

line(s) of visual acuity reference to Snellen visual acuity measurement, in which the notation for distance visual acuity ranges from very low (20/200) to "normal" (20/20) and corresponds to lines of letters of diminishing size on the test chart; for example, a change from 20/20 to 20/30 visual acuity would be described as a "one-line loss," a change from 20/30 to 20/60 would be a "three-line loss," etc.

lipid layer outer layer of the tear film consisting of oily secretions produced in the meibomian glands; see also **tear film**

loop see **lens loop**

loupe low-power magnifying device for viewing objects at very close range; usually referring to two such devices attached to a frame, employed by professionals performing close work on small objects (jeweler's loupes) or by low-vision patients; before the operating microscope came into wide use, the patient's eye would be viewed during surgery through loupes worn by the surgeon

low-tension glaucoma see **glaucoma**

low vision visual impairment that cannot be remedied with corrective lenses or surgical intervention, usually describing a condition in which bilateral retinal pathology (macular degeneration, for example) renders an individual unable to perform normal daily functions; low vision is not synonymous with legal blindness: low vision has no objective definition because people have such widely varying needs for near versus distance vision or the ability to discern colors or fine detail

low vision aids general term for devices designed to help low-vision patients perform their daily tasks; see **bioptics, loupe, magnifier, telescope** and **typoscope**

lumen 1. general term for the hollow area inside a duct or tube (for example, the lumen of the lacrimal duct); 2. in optics, the standard unit of the amount of light flowing through a solid angle (that is, a space shaped like a cone); one lumen (1 lm) is defined as the flux of light through one steradian emitted by a light source with one candle intensity

Mm

macrophthalmia, -os state in which the eyeball is abnormally large

macropia, -sia visual defect in which objects appear larger than they really are

macula general anatomic term derived from the Latin for spot or stain; most commonly in ophthalmic usage, the small yellowish area of the retina where rod and cone cells are most densely packed (more properly called the macula lutea); it is usually centered just below and temporal to the optical axis, is slightly depressed from the surrounding retina, and has at its center the fovea centralis; **corneal m.** area of cloudiness or white opacity on the cornea; **false m.** area of the retina in a nonfixating eye that has an anomalous retinal correspondence with the macula of the fixating eye

macular corneal edema swelling of the cornea accompanied by areas of cloudiness or white opacities

macular degeneration general term for common conditions in which the macula is affected by edema (swelling due to build-up of water in tissue) and dispersion of pigment, resulting in a loss of vision in the center of the field of view; the visual loss is irreversible, although laser treatment and other surgical therapies are employed to slow the progression of macular degeneration; **age-related m.d.** macular degeneration resulting from age-related changes in the small blood vessels, nerve cells pigment epithelium and other tissues in the macula; **dry m.d.** relatively mild form of macular degeneration that is not accompanied by the formation of retinal exudates and is responsible for only a small percentage of cases of vision loss from macular degeneration; **senile m.d.** see **age-related m.d.; wet m.d.** more severe form of macular degeneration that is accompanied by the formation of retinal exudates as a result of new blood vessel growth (choroidal neovascularization) and is responsible for most cases of vision loss from macular degeneration

macular hole appearance of a small, well-defined opening in the macula through the entire depth of the retina, possibly as a result of pulling of the vitreous body on its attachments in the area of the macula

macular pucker see **epiretinal membrane**

macular sparing condition in which the macula is the only functional area of the retina remaining after extensive damage, resulting in a very small area of vision in the center of the visual field

macular splitting visual field defect in which the entire left or right side of the field, including the central area, is lost as a result of damage to the nerve fibers carrying visual impulses from the optic chiasm to the brain

maculopathy general term for diseases of the macula

Maddox rod a transparent rod that is used to change a point source of light into a streak, used in testing visual fusion

magnifier in ophthalmic usage, a device used by low-vision patients to enlarge objects for better viewing, usually to facilitate reading and writing; **hand-held m.** magnifier consisting of high-power plus lens which is held by the user; **projection m.** magnifier that projects an enlarged image of the object to be viewed onto a screen; **stand m.** magnifier consisting of high-power plus lens which is mounted on a stand, leaving the user's hands free

malar bone another name for the zygomatic bone, one of the bones of the orbit

malignant glaucoma see **glaucoma**

malignant myopia see **myopia**

malprojection visual defect in which objects in an image are referred to points in space to which they do not actually correspond; see also **projection**

manifest refraction 1. act of determining the refractive error at distance vision so that the eye does not accommodate, but without using drugs that actually prevent accommodation; 2. the refractive error measured in this manner

manual vitrectomy see **vitrectomy**

Marcus Gunn pupil impairment of the normal response of the pupils to bright light (constriction of both pupils) when either one is stimulated by the light; verified by the swinging flashlight test, in which the examiner shines a light first into one eye, then into the other, then again into the first to discover if the stimulus to one eye results in less constriction than does the same stimulus in the fellow eye; Marcus Gunn pupil appears as a constriction of both pupils when one eye is illuminated, followed by an apparent dilation of both pupils when the fellow eye is illuminated

mast cell cell (present in various tissues including those of the eye) whose exact function is unknown but which plays a role in the release of histamine and other substances involved in inflammation; **m.c. stabilizer** in ophthalmic usage, a topical drug whose action is to prevent mast cells from playing their normal role in the release of histamines and thus prevent or diminish the severity of ocular allergies

maxillary bone one of the bones of the orbit

medial general anatomic term describing a structure or process appearing or occurring in the middle; in ophthalmic usage, referring to the area of the eye nearest the nose; see also **nasal**; compare **lateral** and **temporal**

medial angle see **medial canthus**

medial canthus area where the upper and lower eyelids join at the side of the face nearest the nose; also called the medial canthus and medial angle; compare **lateral canthus**

medial rectus muscle extraocular muscle lying along the side of the eye near the nose and responsible for adducting the eye

medium, -ia in optical usage, substance(s) through which light travels; the fact that light travels at different speeds in different substances accounts for the different degrees to which light is bent (refracted) by various media; see also **refractive index; dioptric m., ocular m.** or **refracting m.** tissues in the eye though which light is transmitted: the cornea, aqueous humor, lens and vitreous humor

megalophthalmia, -os see **macrophthalmia**

megalopia, -sia see **macropia**

meibomian cyst inflammation of the eyelid that results in the collection of fluid within the meibomian glands; see also **chalazion** and **hordeolum**

meibomian glands glands located within the eyelids that produce oily secretions that form the outer layer of the tear fluid layer, also called the **tarsal glands**

meibomianitis or **meibomitis** inflammation of the meibomian glands

melting see **corneal melting**

membrane general medical term for a thin tissue layer that acts as a "skin" or covering, lining or connection between tissues, either as part of normal anatomy or a disease process; **anterior basal m.** see **Bowman's membrane; anterior hyaloid m.** see **hyaloid membrane; basement m.** general medical term for the thin membrane that lies underneath the epithelium of certain tissues, in ophthalmic practice referring to the basement membrane of the choroid and corneal epithelium; see also **Bruch's m., choroidal neovascular m. cyclitic m., Descemet's m., epiretinal m., hyaloid m.,** and **preretinal m.**

membranectomy surgical removal of a membrane, in ophthalmic usage usually referring to removal of retinal membranes

meniscus lens see **convexoconcave lens**

meridian geometric term for a line drawn from one side of a circle or one pole of a sphere to a point diametrically opposite; in ophthalmic usage, one of several standard reference lines used to describe positions on the eyeball

meropia general term for a partial loss of vision

meshwork see **trabecular meshwork**

mesopia vision under conditions of partial lighting, such as dimly lit rooms or outdoors at sunset and sunrise; compare **photopia** and **scotopia**

methylcellulose organic compound that is a component of some artificial tears and viscoelastic substances

microkeratome in ophthalmic usage, device for making thin cuts across the surface of the cornea, creating a thin "button" of flap or corneal tissue as part of a refractive surgical procedure; see also **keratomileusis** and **keratoplasty**

microphthalmia, -os state in which the eye is abnormally small

micropia, -sia visual defect in which objects appear smaller than they really are

microsaccades extremely fine involuntary movements of the eye that occur while the eye is fixated on an object

microscope optical instrument that uses lenses to magnify objects; **operating m.** in ophthalmic surgery, microscope that is used by the surgeon to obtain an enlarged view of the eye; it is typically outfitted with a bright light that shines on the eye and often has multiple eyepieces for use by the assistant surgeon or other personnel, or attachment of a camera

microstrabismus see **strabismus**

minus 1. property of an optical system such that it causes rays of light to diverge (for example, a biconcave lens); 2. in spoken ophthalmic usage, synonym for myopia (for example, a "minus two diopter patient")

minus lens lens that causes incoming rays of light to diverge (see **concave lens**); in common ophthalmic usage, the power of the minus lens used to correct nearsightedness is often used to describe the degree of myopia (thus one hears of a "high minus" or "minus six" patient)

miosis constriction of one or both pupils, physiologically in response to stimulus by bright light or accommodation but also in response to certain drugs or disease processes; compare **mydriasis**

miotic 1. state in which one or both pupils are constricted; 2. any process or agent that constricts the pupils (as in a miotic drug)

mire general term for a reference line of standard shape on a measuring device; see also **keratoscopy**

mixed astigmatism see **astigmatism**

Miyake photography or **view** method for viewing the anterior segment of a cadaver eye from the rear by dissecting the front part of the eye and fixing it to a clear plate, behind which the camera is located

model eye see **schematic eye**

modulation transfer function laboratory method for determining the light-transmitting characteristics of an optical system by analyzing light of known wave form after it passes through the system

Molteno implant or **valve** device implanted to control intraocular pressure by allowing aqueous fluid to drain from the anterior chamber

monochromatism inability to distinguish any colors at all, every object in the field of view appearing in shades of gray ("color blindness")

monocular literally, "one eyed"; used alone to describe a patient with one eye or combined with another term to describe an ocular condition involving only one eye, as in monocular vision (seeing with only one eye), monocular diplopia (double image in one eye), etc.

morgagnian cataract see **cataract**

motor fusion see **fusion**

mucin protein that is the primary component of mucus; in the eye, goblet cells in the conjunctiva produce the mucin that is found in tear fluid

Mueller's cells retinal cells located in the inner nuclear layer with fibers extending to the internal and external limiting membranes; Mueller's cells serve as part of the structural meshwork of the retina and supply nutrients and other metabolic materials to retinal nerve cells

Müller's muscle 1. most commonly in ophthalmic usage, the innermost ring of the ciliary muscle, which functions in accommodation; 2. either of the muscles that keep the upper and lower eyelids from closing

multifocal lens artificial lens that is designed to provide more than one, and usually more than two, focal points; several multifocal systems have been developed for intraocular lenses and contact lenses; see also **aspheric, bifocal lens** and **diffractive multifocal lens**

multiple vision general term for visual defect in which a single object is perceived as several images; see also **diplopia**

mutton-fat precipitates see **keratic precipitates**

mydriasis dilation of one or both pupils, usually as a response to insufficient light but also in response to certain drugs or disease processes; see also **dilation;** compare **miosis**

mydriatic condition or agent that dilates the pupils, as in a mydriatic drug

myope individual with myopia

myopia nearsightedness: refractive error in which the eye focuses rays of light so that the focal point is in front of the retina, with the result that the eye is not able to see objects that are far away; **axial m.** nearsightedness attributable to the length of the eye, that is, the eye is too long for images to be focused on the retina; **degenerative m.** nearsightedness attributable to severe, ongoing structural changes in the eye, eventually resulting in permanent damage to the retina; **high m.** nonspecific term for extreme myopia beyond what is found in most of the population, usually referring to myopia of -6 diopters or greater; **lenticular m.** nearsightedness attributable to excessive power of the lens of the eye, that is, the lens is so powerful it focuses images in front of the retina; **low m.** nonspecific term for small amount of myopia, usually referring to myopia of -2 diopters or less; **malignant m.** see **degenerative m.; moderate m.** nonspecific term referring to an amount of myopia that causes significant but not extreme visual impairment if not corrected, usually referring to myopia between -2 and -6 diopters; **progressive m.** nearsightedness that continues to worsen; **refractive m.** nearsightedness that is attributable to the refractive power of the eye, that is, the refractive power of the cornea and lens is too great and brings incoming rays of light to focus in front of the retina (compare

axial m.); **school m.** nearsightedness that arises from prolonged use of near vision for reading during the school year

myopic keratomileusis see **keratomileusis**

Nn

nanophthalmia, -os see **microphthalmia**

narrow-angle glaucoma see **closed-angle glaucoma** under **glaucoma**

nasal general anatomic term for structure or process that appears or occurs near the nose; see also **medial;** compare **lateral** and **temporal**

nasal bone either of two bones lying between the orbits and forming the bridge of the nose

nasal canthus see **medial canthus**

nasal step glaucoma damage near the central portion of the nasal side of the retina that results in a visual field defect in one quadrant of the temporal visual field (because the damaged retinal fibers actually carry nerve impulses from the temporal retina); the visual field test shows a two-part defect that "steps" from a nasal defect to a temporal one with a normal field in between

nasolacrimal duct canal through which tear fluid drains from the lacrimal sac into the nasal passages; see also **lacrimal apparatus**

near point of accommodation nearest point upon which an eye can focus by accommodation; the greatest degree of accommodation that an eye can attain

near point of convergence nearest point upon which the eyes can maintain binocular vision by convergence; the greatest degree of convergence that the eyes can attain

nearsightedness inability to see distant objects; see **myopia**

near vision vision of objects close to the eye; the distance at which visual tasks such as reading are performed, generally defined to be about 20 cm (8 inches); compare **distance vision**

neovascular glaucoma see **glaucoma**

nerve fiber layer layer of the macula in which retinal nerve cells converge to form the optic nerve; it is the area of the retina that shows early signs of damage in glaucoma; see also **retina**

neuro-ophthalmology medical subspecialty concerned with the optic nerve and the structures of the brain involved in vision

neutralization 1. in optics, act of determining the power of an unknown lens by placing lenses of known opposite powers (that is, minus versus plus lenses) adjacent to the unknown lens and moving the two lenses perpendicular to the line of sight; when there is no motion of a distant object observed through the two lenses, the unknown lens is neutralized and is determined to be the same magnitude but opposite power of the known lens; 2. in retinoscopy, act of determining the refractive state of the eye being examined by adjusting the retinoscope until the pupil is uniformly illuminated regardless of the motion of the retinoscope (because a similar refractive state as with the lenses described definition 1 exists); 3. act of placing corrective lenses or (more commonly) prisms of various powers in front of the eye until any refractive error or strabismus present is corrected

nictitation blinking, especially in animals that have a thin, translucent membrane (nictitating membrane) instead of fleshy eyelids

night blindness see **nyctalopia**

night vision see **scotopia**

nocturnal amblyopia see **amblyopia**

nodal point see **optical center**

no light perception vision total blindness; see also **count-finger vision, hand-motion vision, light perception vision** and **visual acuity**

nonaccommodative esotropia see **esotropia**

nonconcomitant see **incomitant**

noncontact tonometer instrument that measures intraocular pressure without actually touching the eye; see also **pneumotonometer** under **tonometer**

nondominant eye the eye that is subjectively less preferred for use by an individual, much like the way one hand is less preferred than the other; compare **dominant eye**

nuclear adhesions small areas in which the nucleus and cortex of the crystalline lens normally are attached

nuclear cataract see **cataract**

nuclear layer of the retina one of two layers of retinal nerve tissue; the outer nuclear (or bacillary) layer consists of the rod and cone cells, and the inner layer consists of the amacrine and bipolar cells, as well as the capillaries that carry blood through the retina; see also **retina**

nucleus general term for a central structure; in ophthalmic usage, most commonly referring to the nucleus of the crystalline lens

nyctalope individual with nyctalopia

nyctalopia visual defect in which vision is greatly reduced in low light conditions, most often as a result of retinal pigment insufficiency, commonly called "night blindness"

nystagmus condition in which rapid, rhythmic, involuntary eye movements occur; nystagmus is classified according to the type of motion (such as vertical or lateral nystagmus) and the stimuli that cause it to occur; **amaurotic n.** nystagmus of a blind eye; **caloric n.** nystagmus that results when warm or cold fluid is introduced into the ear; **conjugate n.** nystagmus in which the eyes move in their typical parallel fashion; **disjunctive n.** nystagmus in which the eyes move a similar amount but in opposite directions (for example, both eyes turn in toward the nose or out toward the temples); **dissociated n.** nystagmus in which the eyes move independently rather than in their typical parallel fashion; **endpoint n.** nystagmus that occurs when the eyes are turned as far in one direction (up, down, left or right) as possible; **essential n.** nystagmus resulting from some prolonged, unusual use of the eyes (for example, in certain occupations); **fixation n.** nystagmus that occurs after prolonged fixation of the eyes; **jerky n.** see **rhythmic n.; labyrinthine n.** see **caloric n.; latent n.** nystagmus that occurs only when one eye is covered; **rhythmic n.** pattern of slow movement of the eyes in one direction followed by a rapid movement back to the original position; **rotatory n.** nystagmus in which the eyes move in circles; **vestibular n.** see **caloric n.**

Oo

objective lens in optical systems, especially telescopes and microscopes, the lens nearest to the object being viewed; compare **ocular**

oblique astigmatism see **astigmatism**

oblique illumination in slit lamp biomicroscopy, method of visualizing relative depth of ocular structures (for example, cornea, iris and lens) by shining light from the slit lamp light source upon the eye at an angle from the observer's line of sight through the eyepiece; compare **tangential illumination**

oblique muscles see **inferior oblique muscle** and **superior oblique muscle**

O'Brien block injection of anesthetic agents to achieve akinesia (prevention of movement) of the eyelids

occluder instrument used to cover one eye during ophthalmic testing

occlusion general term for blockage or closing; in most common ophthalmic usage, covering an eye, typically during a vision examination; also used in surgery to refer to the blockage of the aspiration port of an irrigation and aspiration probe by tissue that the surgeon wishes to remove

ocul- combining form meaning *eye*

ocular 1. general anatomic adjective meaning of or related to the eye (for example, ocular testing, ocular surgery, etc.); 2. eyepiece of a microscope or other optical instrument; compare **objective lens**

ocular adnexa see **adnexa**

ocular angle see **canthus**

ocular hypertension high intraocular pressure (IOP); IOP of 20 millimeters of mercury (mm Hg) is generally considered the border between low or "normal" IOP and ocular hypertension in otherwise normal eyes; ocular hypertension is not the same as glaucoma, because glaucoma only exists if there is some indication of damage (for example, visual field loss or optic disk cupping) at the current IOP

ocularist individual trained to make and fit ocular prostheses

ocular media tissues in the eye though which light is transmitted: the cornea, aqueous humor, lens and vitreous humor

ocular motility general term for the processes by which the eyes move in a controlled, coordinated fashion, or the study of the function and disorders of alignment and movement of the eyes

ocular pemphigoid see **pemphigoid**

ocular prosthesis artificial device resembling the eye that is placed in the orbit after surgical removal of the eye (correct clinical term for "glass eye"); compare **orbital implant**

oculist archaic term for a medical doctor specializing in care of the eye

oculi uterque Latin phrase meaning either or both eyes, abbreviation for which (OU) is commonly used in ophthalmic speech and literature

oculogyria circular motion ("rolling") of the eyes

oculogyric spasm condition in which the eyes become fixed in an upward gaze

oculomotor general term referring to eye movement and the muscle and nerve systems that initiate and control it

oculomotor nerve the third cranial nerve, which innervates the extraocular muscles

oculopathy general term for unhealthy condition of the eye

oculoplastics surgical specialty concerned with reconstructive and cosmetic surgery of the orbit, eyelids and ocular adnexa

oculopupillary reflex dilation of the pupils when the surface of the eyeball or eyelids are touched or irritated

oculus dexter Latin phrase meaning right eye, abbreviation for which (OD) is commonly used in ophthalmic speech and literature

oculus sinister Latin phrase meaning left eye, abbreviation for which (OS) is commonly used in ophthalmic speech and literature

onchocerciasis condition in which a small parasitic worm infests the skin, connective tissues and eyes of its host; a significant cause of blindness in areas of the world where clean water is not always available; also known as river blindness; see also **filariasis**

-op-, -opt- combining form meaning *see* or *sight*

open-angle glaucoma see **glaucoma**

open-sky general term for surgical procedures (usually vitrectomy) in which the whole cornea is removed to give the surgeon access to the internal structures of the eye; this very traumatic approach has been abandoned in most contemporary ophthalmic surgery

operating microscope see **microscope**

operculated retinal hole or **tear** retinal hole in which a piece of retinal tissue is separated around its entire circumference and pulled away from the surrounding retina by its attachment to the vitreous body

ophthalm- combining form meaning *eye*

ophthalmalgia eye pain

ophthalmia general term for inflammation of the eye; see also **sympathetic ophthalmia**

ophthalmic related to or involving the eye; for example, ophthalmic surgery or ophthalmic disease

ophthalmic artery main vessel bringing blood into the eye and orbit, entering the optic foramen and dividing into vessels that enter the retina, lacrimal apparatus, extraocular muscles, etc.

ophthalmitis general term for inflammation of the eye

ophthalmodynamometry technique for measuring blood pressure in the central retinal artery by applying pressure to the sclera until the artery can be seen retinoscopically to stop pulsating

ophthalmologist medical doctor (MD degree from an accredited medical school) specializing in care of the eye, almost always with certification from the American Board of Ophthalmology; there are currently some 16,000 ophthalmologists in the US, the majority of whom perform surgery as at least part of their practice and belong to the American Academy of Ophthalmology

ophthalmometer general term for any instrument that measures the state of the eye; most commonly in ophthalmic usage referring to a keratometer

ophthalmopathy general term for disease of the eye

ophthalmoplegia paralysis of the eye

ophthalmoscope instrument for viewing the inside of the eye; **binocular o.** ophthalmoscope that allows the examiner to use both eyes when viewing a subject's eye, thereby obtaining a three-dimensional image; see also **direct ophthalmoscopy** and **indirect ophthalmoscopy**

opsoclonia involuntary, arrhythmic movements of the eyes, usually resulting from injury or insult to the brain

optic 1. related to or involving vision or the eye (for example, optic nerve); 2. an element of an optical system (for example, a lens or prism); 3. the central focusing portion of an intraocular lens; compare **haptic**

optical related to or involving a system through which light is transmitted

optical axis see **axis**

optical center point of a lens through which a ray of light may pass without being bent (refracted); also called the nodal point of a lens

optical zone area of a lens or tissue through which the eye sees; used in describing corrective spectacle, contact or intraocular lenses to distinguish the optically functioning part of the lens as distinguished from structural or other parts and in corneal refractive surgery to describe the portion of the cornea that is intended to provide the refractive correction

optic atrophy degeneration of nerve fibers in the optic disk, described in its two major manifestations as primary and secondary optic atrophy

optic chiasm point at which the two optic nerves cross on their path to the brain; in general terms, the impulses from the right and left sides of the retina of each eye are directed to the geniculate body of the brain in such a way that the right brain receives and fuses the right sides of the two retinal images and the left brain receives the left sides

optic cup see **cup**

optic disk roughly circular area of the retina where nerve fibers converge to form the optic nerve, creating an area where images are not perceived; see also **physiologic scotoma** under **scotoma**

optic foramen opening in the orbit (eye socket of the skull) through which the optic nerve passes

optician individual trained to make vision correcting lenses and adjust eyewear

opticist individual specializing in the study of optics

optic nerve one of two bundles of nerve fibers joining each retina to the geniculate body of the brain; the optic nerves meet at the **optic chiasm**

optic nerve head see **optic disk**

opticokinetic relating to the movement of the eyes

optics study of the nature and behavior of light; for important optical principles, see **electromagnetic spectrum, focus, lens, light, prism, reflection** and **refraction**

optometrist doctor of optometry (OD degree from an accredited school of optometry) trained in the diagnosis and treatment of refractive errors and medical conditions of the eye, with some training in general medical principles; most of the 33,000 or so optometrists in the US belong to the American Optometric Association and are authorized (depending on their state's optometric practice laws) to use some prescription pharmaceuticals in diagnosis and treatment of ocular conditions; with very few highly controversial exceptions, no state authorizes optometrists to perform any type of surgery, including laser surgery

optotype general term for standardized image used in visual acuity tests (derived from Snellen's term for the letters on his original chart)

ora serrata irregular anterior border of the retina where it attaches to the choroid, located adjacent to the pars plana of the ciliary body and approximately 8 mm posterior to the corneoscleral limbus

orb in ophthalmic usage, the eyeball

orbicularis muscle muscle controlling the movement of the eyelids and adjacent areas of the face

orbit either of two spherical hollows in the skull that protect and provide attachments for the eyes, extraocular muscles and surrounding tissues; commonly known as the "eye socket," the orbit consists of the ethmoid, frontal, lacrimal, maxillary, palatine, sphenoid and zygomatic bones

orbital crest area of the skull just above the orbit at the level of the eyebrow

orbital decompression surgical procedure to remove bone from the wall of the orbit and thus relieve pressure on the eye, usually in treatment of ocular tumor

orbital fissure one of two openings (superior and inferior) in each orbit through which blood vessels and nerves pass

orbital implant biologically inert device implanted after the contents of the orbit have been surgically removed; compare **ocular prosthesis**

orthokeratology treatment of refractive error by prescribing contact lenses designed to reshape the cornea; often abbreviated ortho-K

orthophoria normal state in which the eyes remain properly oriented even if one or the other is occluded; compare **heterophoria**

orthoptics system for nonsurgical correction of strabismus and other defects of ocular motility; see also **vision training**

oscillating vision state in which objects appear to move back and forth; see also **nystagmus**

osmotic general chemical term for a process or agent that influences the flow of liquids across a membrane; in ophthalmic usage, osmotics are used topically or systemically to draw water out of the eye, thus reducing intraocular pressure

outer granular or **molecular layer of retina** cell layer within the retina where the synapses of the outer and inner nuclear layers meet; see also **retina**

outer limiting membrane of retina see **external limiting membrane of retina**

outer nuclear layer of retina cell layer within the retina composed primarily of bipolar cells and containing the rod and cone cell bodies, located between the inner and outer molecular layers; see also **retina**

outflow in ophthalmic usage, the drainage either of tears through the puncta into the nasolacrimal system or of aqueous humor from the anterior chamber into Schlemm's canal

overcorrection excessive correction of refractive error making a nearsighted eye farsighted or a farsighted eye nearsighted, usually referring to a refractive surgical procedure or intraocular lens implantation that misses its intended target

over-refraction technique of determining the amount of corrective power needed in addition to the corrective lenses currently in place; determined by conducting visual acuity tests while the patient wears eyeglasses or contact lenses

Pp

pachymetry measurement of the thickness of the cornea

palatine bone one of the bones of the orbit

pallor general term for abnormal whiteness (paleness) of tissue; in ophthalmic usage, change in color of the optic disk from yellow to white, indicative of retinal damage (as in glaucoma)

palpebra proper medical term for the eyelid (plural: palpebrae); **inferior p.** lower eyelid; **superior p.** upper eyelid

palpebral conjunctiva ocular tissue comprising the inner surface of the eyelids; compare **bulbar conjunctiva**

palpebral fissure the gap between the upper and lower eyelids

pannus in ophthalmic usage, condition in which blood vessels grow into the cornea, which then becomes fibrous and loses its transparency; may be classified according to type as allergic, glaucomatous, etc.

panophthalmitis widespread inflammation of the tissues of the eye

panretinal photocoagulation laser surgical procedure in which laser energy is applied across wide areas of the retina in an attempt to stop the progression of retinopathy

papilla small nodular elevation on a tissue; plural: papillae; **lacrimal p.** slightly elevated area on the edge of the eyelid, near the nose, where the punctum is located; **optic p.** see **optic disk**

papillae in ophthalmic usage, small elevated areas of palpebral conjunctiva with central blood vessels present in conjunctival infection or allergy

papillary conjunctivitis see **conjunctivitis**

papilledema noninflammatory swelling of the optic disk with engorgement of blood vessels, a result of increased intracranial pressure, malignant hypertension or central retinal vein occlusion; also called **choked disk**

papillomacular bundle dense oval bundle of retinal nerve ganglion cell fibers extending from the macula into the central optic nerve

paracentesis general term for a surgical technique that involves an incision into a fluid-filled cavity; in ophthalmic usage, an incision into the anterior chamber of the eye

paracentral scotoma see **scotoma**

paradoxical general term describing a sign or symptom, such as visual field loss or diplopia, that has a peculiar feature or is of uncertain cause

parakinesia in ophthalmic usage, general term for abnormal movement of the muscles of the eye

parallax optical phenomenon in which an object shifts in the field of view when the observer changes position; objects near to the observer appear to be shifted against a background of distant objects that are more stable; **binocular p.** a shift in the relative position of objects when the observer views first with one eye alone and then with the other eye alone

parophthalmia inflammation of the tissues surrounding the eye

pars general anatomic term meaning part

pars plana commonly used term for the outermost ring of the ciliary body (more properly called the pars plana corporis ciliaris); vitrectomy is sometimes carried out through an incision at the level of the pars plana

pars plicata the innermost ring of the ciliary body, consisting of the ciliary processes

passive forced duction test see **forced duction test**

pemphigoid in ophthalmic usage, a condition in which the conjunctiva blisters, leading to dryness of the eye and adhesion to the eyelids

penetrating keratoplasty surgical procedure in which the entire cornea is removed and replaced with donated tissue, popularly known as corneal transplantation; see also **keratoplasty**

perfluorocarbon class of heavy gases, such as perfluoropropane (C_3F_8), used in retinal detachment repair; see also **gas-fluid exchange**

peribulbar term describing the area around the eye

peribulbar anesthesia anesthesia administered in several injections around the periphery of the eyeball; compare **retrobulbar anesthesia**

perimeter in ophthalmic usage, an instrument that performs perimetry

perimetry technique of visual field testing that determines the boundaries of the field of view by presenting test targets (most often points of light) to the test subject, who fixates upon the middle of a blank screen and reports when the target becomes visible; **automated p.** perimetry in which a machine assists in recording the position of targets and provides a printout of the test results (also called computerized perimetry); **kinetic p.** perimetry in which the targets move from the periphery of the visual field toward the central fixation point until the subject reports that they are visible; **static p.** perimetry in which the targets consist stationary points of light that gradually increase in brightness until the subject reports that they are visible; also see **confrontation field test**

periodic strabismus see **strabismus**

periorbital near the eye or the bony eye socket

peripheral anterior synechiae adhesions between the iris and the cornea

peripheral cataract see **cataract**

peripheral iridectomy see **iridectomy**

peripheral vision perception of objects in the outer areas of the field of view

peritomy in ophthalmic usage, an incision into the conjunctiva

persistence of vision see **afterimage**

phaco- or **phako-** combining form meaning *lens*, usually referring to the natural crystalline lens of the eye but also applicable to artificial lenses; note that in British orthography, phako- is the only acceptable combining form

phaco commonly used abbreviation for phacoemulsification

phacoablation a still-experimental surgical technique of cataract removal by which lens tissue is vaporized by the action of a laser

phacoanaphylaxis condition in which leakage of proteins from the crystalline lens leads to inflammation within the eye

phacodonesis movement of the crystalline lens, usually a result of broken zonules

phacoemulsification surgical technique for cataract extraction using a probe that vibrates at ultrasonic frequency (approximately 40,000 cycles per second) and emulsifies the lens nucleus so that it may be aspirated from the eye through a small incision; **endocapsular p.** technique in which the emulsification of the nucleus is carried out within the area usually enclosed by the lens capsule, which is opened to allow access to the crystalline lens (compare **Kelman p.**); **endolenticular p.** technique in which the emulsification of the nucleus is carried out entirely within the lens capsule and with the lens nucleus remaining in its natural position within the cortex; **intercapsular p.** technique in which the emulsification of the nucleus is carried out through a small slit in the lens capsule; **Kelman p.** original phacoemulsification procedure described by the inventor of phaco, Dr. Charles Kelman, in which the lens nucleus is maneuvered into the anterior chamber and then emulsified; **one-handed p.** general term for techniques of phacoemulsification in which only one instrument (the phaco probe) is used during emulsification of the nucleus; **two-handed p.** general term for techniques in which a second instrument is used by the surgeon to maneuver the lens as it is being emulsified by the phaco probe

phacoerysis obsolete technique for cataract extraction using a suction device

phacolytic glaucoma see **glaucoma**

phakic state in which the natural lens of the eye is in place (compare aphakic)

phako- see **phaco**

phase property of wave energy such that the "peaks" and "troughs" of many individual waves can coincide with each other or cancel each other; waves with peaks and troughs that coincide are said to be in phase; also see **coherent light**

phlyctenular keratoconjunctivitis see **keratoconjunctivitis**

phlyctenule small, fluid-filled blisters that can appear on the conjunctiva, in which case they are accompanied by neovascularization, or on the cornea

phoria general term for movement of one or both eyes out of alignment when fusion is prevented by occlusion of one eye; **horizontal p.** phoria in the horizontal plane; **vertical p.** phoria in the vertical plane; see also **esophoria, exophoria, heterophoria, hyperphoria, hypophoria** and **orthophoria**

phoropter instrument fitted with a number of different types of lenses that are rotated into place in front of a test subject's eyes to determine the amount of vision correction necessary; formerly a brand name for one style of such instrument but now used generically

photo- combining word meaning *light*

photoablation action of the excimer laser to vaporize tissue

photocoagulation in ophthalmic usage, application of laser light that is absorbed by the blood present in ocular tissues, which causes disruption of the cells and formation of scar tissue, which can be therapeutic; see also **laser**

photon smallest unit (sometimes described as a particle or quantum) of light energy

photophobia excessive sensitivity of the eyes to light

photopia daylight vision, in which the rod cells of the retina are suppressed and the cones are the primary light perceiving cells; compare **scotopia**

photopsia appearance of flashes of light in the field of view attributable to some defect of the retina or optic tract

photoreceptors the cells in the retina that transmit nerve impulses when stimulated by light: rod cells and cone cells

photorefractive keratectomy application of the excimer laser to remove corneal tissue in order to change the surface curvature of the eye and thus corrective refractive error

phototherapeutic keratectomy application of the excimer laser to remove corneal tissue in order to treat pathology rather than to change any refractive error of the eye

phototoxicity property of bright light such that it damages the retina upon prolonged exposure

phthisis (pronounced "tie-sis") general term for gradual loss of the bulk and structure of a bodily organ; most commonly in ophthalmic usage referring to phthisis bulbi, in which a blind eye will shrink away, necessitating surgical removal

physiologic astigmatism see **astigmatism**

physiologic blind spot or **scotoma** see **scotoma**

piggyback intraocular lens see **intraocular lens**

pigmentary glaucoma see **glaucoma**

pigment dispersion syndrome condition in which iris pigment is scattered and appears as small deposits on other anterior segment structures; compare **pigmentary glaucoma** under **glaucoma**

pinguecula abnormal growth of yellowish membrane at the junction of the sclera and cornea that can progress to pterygium

pink eye see **conjunctivitis**

Placido disk disk with concentric circles used to evaluate corneal curvature; see also **keratoscopy**

plano lens lens that has no refracting power: rays of light falling straight onto a lens that is piano on both surfaces continue on their straight-line paths; also, a lens may have one convex or concave surface in combination with one plano surface, in which case it is called planoconvex or planoconcave, respectively

platysmal reflex constriction of the pupil in response to manipulation of the platysma, a muscle in the area of the jaw

plica general anatomic term for a fold of tissue

plica ciliaris the small folds of tissue in the ciliary body

plica lacrimalis fold of skin that acts as the valve of the tear gland

plica semilunaris half-moon shaped fold of tissue formed where the nasal portion of the bulbar conjunctiva joins muscle tissue

plus 1. property of an optical system such that it causes rays of light to converge (for example, a biconvex lens); 2. in spoken ophthalmic usage, synonym for hyperopia (for example, a "plus two diopter patient")

plus lens lens that causes rays of light to converge (see **convex lens**); in common ophthalmic usage, the power of the plus lens used to correct farsightedness is often used to describe the degree of hyperopia (thus one hears of a "high plus" or "plus six" patient)

pneumatic retinopexy see **retinopexy**

pneumotonometer see **tonometer**

polar cataract see **cataract**

polarized light light that has been altered so that the normally random planes of its transverse wave motions (that is, the plane in which the theoretical "peaks" and "troughs" lie) are aligned along the same pole; polarizing filters are used in various optical instruments and also in some types of sunglasses

polycarbonate lightweight, shatter-resistant polymer used as a spectacle lens material

polycoria condition in which there appears to be more than one pupillary opening in the iris

polymegethism in ophthalmic usage, condition in which corneal endothelial cells become irregular in size and shape; note that this spelling is based on authorities' citation of Greek *poly* ("many") being joined with *megethos* ("size") rather than *megalos* ("large")

polymethylmethacrylate acrylic polymer used in the manufacture of contact lenses ("hard lenses") and intraocular lenses

polyopia, -sia, -y general term for visual defect in which one object appears as multiple images; see also **diplopia**

polypropylene flexible polymer used in the manufacture of sutures and some intraocular lens haptics

posterior capsulotomy see **capsulotomy**

posterior chamber portion of the eye behind the crystalline lens-zonule apparatus and ciliary body, containing the vitreous humor and retinal tissues; compare **anterior chamber**

posterior chamber intraocular lens see **intraocular lens**

posterior hyaloid membrane see **hyaloid membrane**

posterior pole of the eye imaginary point at the rear surface of the sclera directly opposite the anterior pole of the eye

posterior pole of the lens point at the rear and center of the crystalline lens; compare **anterior pole of the lens**

posterior segment of the eye general term describing the structures of the eye lying behind the lens-zonule apparatus and ciliary body; ophthalmic surgery is roughly divided into the categories of anterior segment (cornea, glaucoma and cataract procedures) and posterior segment (retina and vitreous procedures)

posterior staphyloma see **staphyloma**

posterior subcapsular cataract see **cataract**

posterior toric method of stabilizing toric contact lenses by incorporating the toric optics into the posterior surface of the lens, theoretically achieving a shape complementary to that of the cornea, helping to prevent rotation and maintain the orientation of the lens to correct astigmatism in the proper axis; compare **dynamic stabilization, prism ballast** and **truncation**

posterior vitreous detachment separation of the vitreous body from its normal attachment to the retina, usually following syneresis (degenerative shrinking of the vitreous) but sometimes as a result of trauma; symptoms include flashers and floaters, and posterior vitreous detachment sometimes causes retinal breaks, as the posterior vitreous is firmly attached to the retina; abbreviation: PVD

potential acuity visual acuity that theoretically could be attained in an eye if all correctable defects (usually referring to opacities of normally clear refractive ocular media) were corrected

Prentice's law optical formula defining the amount that a ray of light deviates (measured in prism diopters, Δ) from its original straight path when passing through a point a given distance (measured in centimeters, cm) from the center of a lens of a given power (measured in diopters, D), expressed as $\Delta = D \times cm$

preretinal membrane condition in which a membrane forms between the retina and the vitreous humor in the region of the macula

presbyope individual with presbyopia

presbyopia naturally occurring process of aging whereby changes in ocular tissues result in loss of accommodation in near vision, usually occurring soon after 40 years of age

primary occurring initially, that is, before a secondary condition, procedure, etc., but not necessarily causing it; compare **secondary;** for entities described as primary, look up entry under main word, such as: **primary glaucoma** see **glaucoma,** etc.

primary deviation strabismus in which one eye deviates from its position of fixation when the fellow eye fixates; compare **secondary deviation**

principal axis see **axis**

prism general term for a transparent object having at least two flat surfaces at an angle to each other (most commonly a triangle in cross section), that bends light rays from their original path but allows them to continue traveling in parallel paths (compare **lens**); also, any component of an optical system that functions as a prism (for example, the degree to which a concave spectacle lens is thicker around the edges than in the center, bending light more in the periphery of the lens); **base-down, base-in, base-out** and **base-up p.** description of the orientation of prisms in front of the eye, prescribed to diagnose and/or correct various types of strabismus (for example, base-in prisms bend light rays so that objects appear to be further out from the center of the field of view than they really are); also, when a prismatic component is prescribed in a spectacle lens, the possible orientations are described as base-in, etc. (base-in prism, for example, is prescribed to achieve greater refractive power when the eyes are convergent in near vision)

prism angle angle at which the two refracting surfaces of a prism meet

prism apex line formed by the junction of the refracting surfaces of a prism

prism ballast method of stabilizing toric contact lenses by thickening the bottom with prism power, thereby making the bottom of the lens heavier and/or the top of the lens less resistant to the mechanical action of the lids during blinking, which helps prevent rotation and maintain the orientation of the lens to correct astigmatism in the proper axis; compare **dynamic stabilization, posterior toric** and **truncation**

prism bar device in which prisms of increasing power are arranged in a row so that they can be easily moved one after another in front of the eye in examining the alignment of the eyes; can be either a **horizontal p.b.** or a **vertical p.b.**

prism base flat surface of a prism opposite the apex

prism diopter measure of the refracting power of a prism, or the prismatic effect of a lens, in which one prism diopter (abbreviation: Δ) is defined as the power that deflects a ray of light 1 centimeter from its original path measured at a point 1 meter from the prism; see also **diopter** and **Prentice's law**

progressive addition lens spectacle lens (often referred to as *progressive adds* or simply *progressives*) in which the refractive power increases from the center toward the periphery to provide a range of correction from far to near; used in the correction of presbyopia to avoid visible lines on the lens as seen with bifocal or trifocal lenses

progressive cataract see **cataract**

progressive myopia see **myopia**

projection in ophthalmic usage, process by which objects in an image are mentally connected to various points in space; **anomalous p.** mental connection of an image to a point in space by processes other than those that occur in normal, healthy visual systems (see also **anomalous retinal correspondence**); **erroneous p.** visual defect in which objects in an image are referred to points in space to which they do not actually correspond

prolapse general term for shifting of an anatomic structure out of its normal position and through another structure; also see **iris prolapse**

proliferative vitreoretinopathy see **retinopathy**

proptosis protruding eyeball

protanomaly impairment of ability to distinguish shades of red and green

protanopia severe inability to distinguish shades of red and green

provocative test general term for test in which the examiner attempts to elicit an abnormal response to a stimulus (provoking high intraocular pressure, for example, when glaucoma is suspected)

pseudoaccommodation ability to see to some degree at both near and distance when true accommodation is impossible (either because of the onset of presbyopia or in some other circumstance); used to describe range of vision achieved, for example, when a monofocal intraocular lens is implanted in an eye with a low degree of astigmatism

pseudoesophoria and **pseudoexophoria** deviations of an eye inward or outward, respectively, attributable to some temporary extraocular condition; compare **esophoria** and **exophoria**

pseudoexfoliation syndrome appearance of dark deposits, which appear to be iris pigment but are not, on structures of the anterior chamber; compare **exfoliation**

pseudomyopia temporary condition of nearsightedness created when spasm of the ciliary muscle puts the eye in a state of accommodation

pseudophakia state in which an intraocular lens is present in the eye

pseudophakic bullous keratopathy see **keratopathy**

pseudophakos see **intraocular lens**

pseudopsia visual hallucination

pseudopterygium see **pterygium**

pseudoptosis apparent drooping of the eyelid that is actually a result of an abnormally small opening between the two eyelids; compare **ptosis**

pseudotumor cerebri increase in intracranial pressure on the brain that is not due to presence of a tumor, resulting in ocular symptoms such as blurred and double vision, swelling of the optic nerve head and strabismus

pseudo-von Graefe's sign failure of the upper eyelid to move downward when the eye is turned downward, attributable to abnormal healing after damage to the nerve fibers connected to the eyelid muscles; compare **von Graefe's sign**

pterygium fully attached triangular membrane of fleshy tissue extending from a base in the conjunctiva of the canthus toward and possibly onto the cornea, sometimes arising from a pinguecula; usually caused by excessive exposure of the eye to irritation (for example, dust, wind and direct sunlight); **cicatricial p.** or **pseudopterygium** triangular adhesion of the conjunctiva to the cornea resembling pterygium but attached only at its apex

ptosis in ophthalmic usage, a drooping of the upper eyelid, sometimes occurring after the eyelid has been stretched by a speculum placed during surgery; **p. adiposa** ptosis caused by deposit of fatty tissue in the upper eyelid; **false p.** see **pseudoptosis**; **Homer's p.** ptosis accompanied by miosis and flushing of the face, caused by a nerve defect; **levator p.** ptosis caused by defect of the levator muscle; **morning**

or **waking p.** normal drooping of the upper eyelid noted upon waking from sleep

puncta plural of **punctum**

punctal occlusion method for treating dry eye syndrome by blocking the outflow of tears through the puncta, either temporarily by inserting a **punctum plug** or permanently by laser surgery

punctum in ophthalmic usage, one of the openings in the eyelids through which tear fluid drains out of the eye; there are one each in the upper (**superior p.**) and lower (**inferior p.**) lids located 2 to 4 mm from the medial canthus; plural: puncta

punctum plug device that is designed to be inserted into (and later removed from) the punctum in order to treat dry eye by blocking the outflow of tears

pupil normally circular opening in the center of the iris that controls the amount of light passing through the eye to the retina by opening (dilating) in dim light in a process called mydriasis and closing (constricting) in bright light in a process called miosis; **fixed p.** see **tonic p.; tonic p.** pupil in which the normal pupillary reflexes are severely diminished or absent; for a number of other unusual states and abnormal conditions of the pupil that are noteworthy, see also **Adie p., Argyll Robertson p., Behr p., cat's eye p., keyhole p.,** and **Marcus Gunn p.**

pupillary axis see **axis**

pupillary block condition in which the iris adheres to the structures behind it, blocking the normal flow of aqueous humor into the anterior chamber and resulting in a build-up of intraocular pressure; see also **iris bombé** and **pupillary block glaucoma** under **glaucoma**

pupillary dilator muscle iris muscle encircling the outer edge of the iris and extending into the ciliary body, responsible for dilating the pupil; compare **pupillary sphincter muscle**

pupillary distance measurement of the distance from the center of one pupil to the center of the pupil of the fellow eye

pupillary margin heavily pigmented area of the iris immediately surrounding the pupil

pupillary muscle see **pupillary sphincter muscle** and **pupillary dilator muscle**

pupillary reflex any one of a number of responses of the pupil to stimulus, usually referring to the reaction of pupil size to varying intensity of light (see details under **pupil**), but also including: **accommodative p.r.** constriction of the pupil in near vision; **consensual p.r.** normal state in which dilation or constriction of one pupil in response to a stimulus is accompanied by a similar response in the pupil of the fellow eye, even if the stimulus is only delivered to one eye; **oculosensory p.r.** or **oculopupillary reflex** dilation of the pupils when the surface of the eyeball or eyelids are touched or irritated

pupillary sphincter muscle iris muscle encircling the pupil, responsible for constricting the pupil; compare **pupillary dilator muscle**

pupillary zone area of the iris adjacent to the pupil

pupilloplasty general term for surgical procedure to alter the appearance or function of the pupil, usually referring to repair of a damaged pupil

pupilloplegia paralysis of the pupil; see also **tonic pupil**

Purkinje images reflections from the surfaces of the cornea and crystalline lens, useful in determining the curvature and relative position of these surfaces in ophthalmoscopy

Purkinje shift change in sensitivity of vision from daylight to dark in which the retina becomes more sensitive to the blue-green part of the electromagnetic spectrum in low light levels; see also **scotopia**

Qq

Q-switched laser see **laser**

quadrantanopia, -opsia partial or total loss of one quarter of the visual field, resulting from some extraocular defect such that the visual fields of both eyes can be affected; **crossed binasal q.** quandrantanopia of the lower nasal portion of one visual field and the upper nasal portion of the other visual field; **crossed bitemporal q.** quadrantanopia of the lower temporal portion of one visual field and the upper temporal portion of the other visual field; **heteronymous q.** quadrantanopia affecting different portions of the two visual fields (for example, the upper temporal region of one and the lower nasal region of the other visual field); **homonymous q.** quadrantanopia affecting similar portions of both visual fields (for example, the upper temporal regions of both visual fields)

quantum fundamental unit of light energy; see also **photon**

Rr

radial keratotomy refractive surgical procedure in which corneal incisions are placed radially, like the spokes of a wheel, in order to flatten the cornea and correct nearsightedness; the degree of flattening depends upon the depth (about 90% of the corneal thickness) and number (typically from four to eight) of incisions; see also **keratotomy**

radian measurement of the size of an angle, defined as the angle that subtends an arc on the circumference of a circle equal to the radius of the circle (equal to approximately 67°)

radiuscope instrument for measuring the curvature of contact lenses

radix general anatomic term for the "root" of a structure, as in the **optic nerve r.,** which joins the optic nerve to the geniculate body of the brain

raphe general anatomic term for junction line between two halves of a structure; **retinal r.** horizontal line in the retinal nerve fiber layer on the temporal side of the macula on either side of which the nerve fibers follow diverging paths to the optic disk

reading vision see **near vision**

rectus muscle see **inferior rectus muscle, internal rectus muscle** and **superior rectus muscle**

recurrent corneal erosion see **corneal erosion**

red-free photography photography of the eye using green ("red-free") light, so structures that would appear red under normal white light appear black, thereby increasing contrast and enhancing images of blood vessels, inflammation and hemorrhages

red reflex reflection of light from the retina, which appears as a bright red area through the pupil upon funduscopy and examination of the eye through the operating microscope

reflection property of light such that it bounces back from the surface of an object or interface between two substances with different indices of refraction; light rays striking the interface are called incident and those bouncing back are called reflected

reflex 1. muscle reaction to stimulation; 2. reflection of light; see also **red reflex**

refract 1. to bend light by refraction (see **refraction,** definition 1); 2. to perform a refraction (see **refraction,** definition 2)

refraction 1. action of the interface between two transparent media such that light is bent from its normal straight-line course when passing from one to the other; see **refractive index;** 2. in ophthalmic practice, the act of determining what power lens is needed to correct an ametropia; see also **over-refraction;** 3. in ophthalmic speech and literature, the power of a lens needed to correct an ametropia is referred to as the refraction of a given individual, leading to informal descriptions such as "the (patient's) refraction was minus two diopters"; see also **manifest refraction**

refractive amblyopia see **amblyopia**

refractive error see **ametropia**

refractive index property of an optical medium defined as the ratio of the velocity of light in air to the velocity of light in the medium (abbreviated N); the change in velocity from one medium to another is proportional to the degree of refraction; materials with a large index of refraction can be fashioned into high-power lenses that are relatively thin, thus avoiding the peripheral distortion caused by thick corrective lenses

refractive keratoplasty corneal surgery performed to corrective refractive error; see also **refractive surgery** and **keratoplasty**

refractive media see **medium**

refractive surgery surgical procedure that has as its primary objective the correction of an ametropia; see also **clear lensectomy, epikeratophakia, excimer laser, intrastromal corneal ring, keratomileusis, keratophakia, keratoplasty, keratotomy** and **thermo-keratoplasty**

refractometry objective measurement of the focusing power of the eye to determine the power of corrective lenses needed without depending upon the patient's perception of visual acuity, used in refraction of very young patients or those unable to participate in subjective refraction; see also **retinoscope**

regression in refractive surgery, phenomenon in which the correction achieved in the immediate postoperative period drifts back toward the original refractive error

regular astigmatism see **astigmatism**

reticule pattern of lines, usually a standardized scale, inscribed in optical instruments to allow the examiner to make quantitative observations of the subject

retina transparent light-sensitive structure lying at the back of the eye between the vitreous body and the choroid; light striking the retina passes through the internal limiting membrane (also known as the posterior hyaloid face of the vitreous); the retinal nerve fiber layer; the ganglion cell layer; the inner molecular and inner nuclear layers which, like the outer molecular and outer nuclear layers just beneath them, are composed of nerve cells and synapses; the external limiting membrane; the bacillary layer (composed of the light-sensitive rod and cone cells); and finally the retinal pigment epithelium (which plays no part in visual sensation but a key role in retinal nutrition), which is attached to the choroid; also see **amacrine cells, bipolar cells, fovea, macula, optic disk** and **ora serrata**

retinal accommodation accommodation induced by perception of an unfocused image on the retina

retinal adaptation process whereby the retina adjusts to the level of light in the environment, becoming more or less sensitive to light under relatively dark and light conditions, respectively

retinal apoplexy condition in which the central retinal vein is blocked, leading to an impairment of the retina's blood supply and eventual damage

retinal artery see **branch** and **central retinal artery**

retinal branch vein occlusion see **branch retinal vein occlusion**

retinal central artery occlusion see **central retinal artery occlusion**

retinal central vein occlusion see **central retinal vein occlusion**

retinal correspondence property of vision such that a point on one retina becomes associated in the brain with a point on the retina of the fellow eye; see **anomalous retinal correspondence** and **harmonious retinal correspondence**

retinal dehiscence see **retinal dialysis**

retinal detachment condition in which the bacillary layer (rod and cone cells) of the retina is partially or completely separated from the pigment epithelial layer, resulting in a loss of vision in the area that is detached; **rhegmatogenous r.d.** retinal detachment that begins as a break or tear in the retina (for example, following trauma to the eye); **tractional r.d.** detachment in which the retina is pulled away from the pigment epithelial layer (for example, as a complication of vitrectomy)

retinal dialysis retinal tear in the area of the ora serrata

retinal dysplasia general term for abnormal development of retinal tissue

retinal exudates light-colored bodies that appear on the retina in a number of retinal conditions, may be either **hard exudates,** which are well-defined yellowish bodies that are truly the result of exudation (leakage of proteins from retinal tissue), or **soft exudates,** which are not exudates at all but small areas of the retinal nerve fiber layer that have lost their blood supply and become wispy white areas with no clear borders, usually appearing in diabetic and other types of retinopathy; see also **cotton-wool spots**

retinal hole see **retinal tear**

retinal ischemia condition in which the blood supply of the retina is cut off, resulting in tissue damage; see also **branch retinal artery** and **vein occlusion, central retinal artery** and **vein occlusion** and **retinal exudates**

retinal pigment epithelium dark, posterior-most layer of the retina, providing attachment to the choroid and important functions in retinal nutrition

retinal recovery see **retinal adaptation**

retinal reflex see **red reflex**

retinal rivalry process in which there is blurring of an area of the visual field when different images are presented to corresponding areas of the two retinae

retinal tear opening in the retina caused by a pull from the vitreous humor, trauma or surgical complication; see also **giant retinal break or tear** and **retinal detachment**

retinal vein see **branch retinal artery** and **central retinal artery**

retinitis general term for inflammation of the retina; **actinic r.** retinitis resulting from exposure to ultraviolet radiation; **central serous r.** inflammation and swelling of the macula with leakage of blood vessels and visual impairment, possibly leading to retinal detachment; **circinate r.** retinitis marked by the appearance of a circle of white patches around the macula, which can lead to retinal hemorrhaging; **cytomegalovirus r.** opportunistic infection of the retina in immunocompromised patients (such as those with AIDS); **diabetic r.** see **diabetic retinopathy; exudative r.** retinitis marked by the appearance of **retinal exudates; purulent r.** retinitis caused by infection in the eye; **serous r.** inflammation of the retina characterized by swelling of the macula

retinitis pigmentosa inherited condition in which deposits of melanin pigment appear on the retina, accompanied by diminishment of retinal blood vessels and pallor of the optic disc, leading eventually to loss of vision

retinoblastoma malignant tumor arising from the retinal cells of an embryo and developing in the first few years of life

retinography photography of the retina

retinopathy general term for abnormal condition of the retina, specifically: **central disciform r.** degeneration of the retina in elderly individuals following a hemorrhage in the macula; **diabetic r.** ocular effect of systemic diabetes mellitus characterized by retinal swelling, multiple small hemorrhages, retinal exudates and growth of blood vessels into the retina, with progressive loss of vision if left untreated; **proliferative (vitreo-) retinopathy** neovascularization of the retina and vitreous in certain conditions involving the circulatory system, such as diabetes mellitus

retinopathy of prematurity condition affecting premature infants who are placed in oxygen-enriched environments, occurring less frequently than in the past now that there is increased awareness of risks; marked by neovascularization of the retina, which is followed by retinal hemorrhage, scarring and occasionally detachment, and growth of fibrous tissue into the vitreous humor; the possibility of serious ocular conditions such as glaucoma is increased following retinopathy of prematurity (the advanced stage of which is also called retrolental fibroplasia)

retinopexy surgical procedure to repair a retinal detachment, most commonly through injection of air or heavy gas following vitrectomy (**pneumatic retinopexy**) or sometimes application of extreme cold to the external globe (**cryoretinopexy**)

retinoschisis splitting of the tissue layers of the retina, usually progressing slower than other types of retinal detachment

retinoscope hand-held instrument that projects a spot or streak of light that is reflected by the retina; the apparent motion of the reflected light when the instrument is moved allows the examiner to determine the refractive state of the eye; see also **refractometry**

retinoscopy technique of objective refractometry using the retinoscope

retinosis general term for abnormal, noninflammatory condition of the retina

retinotomy general term for surgical incision into the retina

retraction syndrome inherited condition marked by mild enophthalmos, inability of the eye to abduct, and partial closure of the eyelids upon adduction

retrobulbar general term describing the area behind the eye

retrobulbar anesthesia anesthesia administered by injection behind the eye; compare **peribulbar anesthesia**

retroillumination method of viewing an ocular structure by reflected light in which the light source is shined upon an ocular structure (often the retina) lying behind the one to be viewed; usually referring to slit lamp biomicroscopy but can also describe a technique used with operating microscopes; see also **indirect illumination**

retrolental term describing the area behind the lens

retrolental fibroplasia see **retinopathy of prematurity**

rhegmatogenous retinal detachment see **retinal detachment**

ribbon keratitis see **keratitis**

rigid gas-permeable lens see **contact lens**

ring keratitis see **keratitis**

ring scotoma see **scotoma**

river blindness see **onchocerciasis**

rod cells one of two types of light-sensitive cells in the retina; often simply referred to as rods, they function primarily in night vision; see also **cone cells** under **cone** and **scotopia**

rosacea keratitis see **keratitis**

rose bengal dye used in ophthalmic applications to stain the surface of the eye and detect damaged or dead conjunctival or corneal epithelial cells

rotatory nystagmus see **nystagmus**

Roth's spots infectious retinitis in which white areas appear in the optic disk surrounded by areas of hemorrhage

rubeosis iridis growth of blood vessels into the iris in individuals with diabetes mellitus or following trauma

Ss

saccade rapid, voluntary movement of the eyes from one point of fixation to another in a series of jerky steps

saccadic fixation rapid change of fixation from one point to another in the visual field

saccadic movement see **saccade**

schematic eye device used in training for retinoscopy; two telescoping cylinders are used to vary the length of the schematic eye (representing the axial length of human eyes) and auxiliary lenses are placed in the anterior segment of the schematic eye to simulate astigmatism and other refractive errors; the examiner places trial lenses in front of the auxiliary lens while viewing the inside of the schematic eye's posterior segment though the retinoscope

Schiotz tonometer see **indentation tonometer** under **tonometer**

Schirmer test test of tear production in which one end of a 5 x 25 mm strip of filter paper is placed inside the eyelid over the inferior lacrimal punctum; wetting of the paper at a rate of 2 to 3 mm per minute is considered normal

Schlemm's canal ring-shaped network of passages in the scleral sulcus through which aqueous humor drains into the bloodstream (fluid is prevented from flowing back into the anterior chamber)

Schwalbe's line border of Descemet's membrane, appearing upon gonioscopy as a dark line at the edge of the cornea

scintillating scotoma see **scotoma**

scirrhophthalmia condition in which a hard malignant tumor appears in the tissues of the eye

sclera the tough, fibrous, light-colored tissue that makes up the major outer layer of the eye (holding the choroid and retina within it), approximately spherical in shape with a small opening posteriorly (the porus opticus) where the optic nerve passes through it and a larger opening anteriorly where it joins with the clear cornea, which is composed of tissue very similar to that of the sclera; **blue s.** appearance of a thin sclera when pigment and blood from underlying tissue (the choroid) gives it a bluish tint

scleral buckling procedure general term for surgical techniques to repair retinal detachment in which a device (such as an elastic band) is used to indent the sclera in the region of the detachment, bringing the pigment epithelium layer back into contact with the bacillary layer of the retina

scleral canal see **Schlemm's canal**

scleral conjunctiva see **conjunctiva**

scleral foramen see **lamina cribrosa**

scleral lens large-diameter contact lens used in orthokeratology and treatment of certain conditions of the external ocular tissues; see also **contact lens**

scleral show excessive exposure of sclera due to abnormally wide opening of the eyelids

scleral spur band of scleral fibers located between Schlemm's canal and the ciliary muscle, serving as part of the anchor tissue for the ciliary muscle

scleral sulcus area where the fibrous tissues of the cornea insert into the similarly fibrous tissues of the sclera

scleral trabeculae see **trabecular meshwork**

sclerectasia, -asis protrusion of the sclera

sclerectomy general term for surgical removal of scleral tissue

scleritis inflammation of the sclera; **anterior s.** scleritis affecting the forward, visible part of the sclera; **necrotizing s.** slowly progressive degeneration of the sclera to the point of perforation, often associated with rheumatoid arthritis; **posterior s.** scleritis affecting the rear, non-visible portion of the sclera and Tenon's capsule

sclerocorneal of or related to the sclera and cornea together

scleromalacia condition marked by thinning and softening of the sclera

scleromalacia perforans see **necrotizing scleritis** under **scleritis**

scleronyxis surgical procedure involving a puncturing of the sclera

scleroplasty general term for surgical procedure on the sclera

sclerostomy general term for the surgical creation of an opening in the sclera, most commonly in an attempt to allow drainage of fluids from the anterior chamber in the treatment of glaucoma

sclerotic scatter in slit lamp biomicroscopy, method of viewing the cornea by shining light from the slit lamp light source upon the corneal limbus; the light will show as a bright ring around the limbus and be refracted throughout corneal tissue to provide a view of its structure and any pathology that might be present

sclerotomy general term for an incision into the sclera

scoto- combining word meaning dark

scotoma area within the visual field in which vision is impaired or absent, attributable to dysfunction of the retina; plural: scotomata; **absolute s.** area within the visual field where there is no vision; **annular s.** ring-shaped scotoma, usually centered on the fixation point; **arcuate s.** scotoma that extends from the physiologic scotoma across the visual field in an arc-like shape (see **Bjerrum's scotoma**); **central s.** scotoma in the center of the visual field corresponding to impairment of function of the macula; **centrocecal s.** egg-shaped scotoma extending from the physiologic scotoma to the fixation point, corresponding to damage across the width of the macula; **color s.** area within the visual field where color vision is impaired or absent; **comet s.** see **arcuate s.; false s.** area of impairment in the visual field that is not attributable to dysfunction of the retina (for example, scotoma caused by a small undiagnosed cataract); **hemianopic s.** scotoma covering half the visual field (see also **hemianopia**); **insular s.** scotoma surrounded by an area of normal vision; **junction s.** scotoma arising from a defect in the optic chiasm (junction of the two optic nerves); **motile s.** type of false scotoma in which opaque material (for example, cells) floating through the vitreous results in the appearance of dark areas within the visual field that shift with the passing of time; **negative s.** scotoma that is unnoticed by the affected individual but demonstrable on visual field testing; **paracentral s.** scotoma attributable to an area of dysfunction near the macula; **pericecal** or **peripapillary s.** scotoma occurring near the physiologic scotoma; **peripheral s.** scotoma that is located well away from the fixation point; **physiologic s.** normally occurring point in the visual field where there is no vision, corresponding to the area of the optic disk where retinal nerve fibers converge to form the optic nerve (also called the physiologic blind spot); **positive s.** scotoma that is noticeable to the affected individual; **quadrantic s.** scotoma involving one quarter of the visual field (see also **quadrantanopia**);

relative s. area of the visual field in which vision is impaired compared with adjacent areas, or diminished response to some visual stimuli (for example, color) but not others; **ring s.** see **annular s.; scintillating s.** scotoma with a jagged outline surrounded by bright flashes, often reported to precede attacks of migraine; **Seidel's s.** progression of arcuate scotoma or enlargement of the physiologic blind spot

scotopia night vision, in which the rod cells of the retina are sensitized with the pigment rhodopsin in the process of dark (scotopic) adaptation; compare **nyctalopia** and **photopia**

secondary occurring after the primary condition, procedure, etc., but not necessarily as a result of it; compare **primary;** for conditions described as secondary, look up entry under main word, such as: **secondary cataract** see **cataract, secondary glaucoma** see **glaucoma,** etc.; follow same approach for devices and procedures, such as: **secondary IOL** see **IOL,** etc.

secondary deviation deviation of the eye that normally fixates in strabismus when the eye that normally does not fixate is forced to do so

sector iridectomy see **iridectomy**

segment term used in opticianry to describe the near vision optical element placed in the lower portion of a corrective bifocal lens; see also **add**

Seidel scotoma see **scotoma**

Seidel sign appearance of aqueous humor leaking from the anterior chamber onto the surface of the eye, possibly revealed by applying pressure to the eye and sometimes enhanced with the use of dyes

semilunar fold flap of conjunctiva normally found near the medial canthus

senile general term meaning old age

senile cataract see **cataract**

senile ectropion ectropion occurring in elderly individuals due to the loss of elasticity of the tissues of the eyelid

senile macular degeneration see **macular degeneration**

sensory fusion merging of the images from the two eyes into a single image by the brain

sensory retina all layers of the retina involved in the perception of light (all layers except the retinal pigment epithelium); see also **retina**

Sherrington's law of reciprocal innervation general principle of physiology, also applicable to the extraocular muscles, that every stimulus inducing a muscle to contract is accompanied by an equal stimulus for the antagonistic muscle (that is, the one with the opposite effect) to relax

siderosis general term for condition in which deposits of iron appear in bodily tissues

siderosis bulbi siderosis within the eye

siderosis conjunctivae deposits of iron in the conjunctiva, usually from a foreign body

silicone contact lens see **contact lens**

silicone IOL see **intraocular lens**

silicone oil heavy fluid used in surgery to repair retinal detachment; see also **gas-fluid exchange**

sine-wave grating vision test target consisting of patterns of lines of various density for which the test subject is asked to describe the orientation (vertical, horizontal, etc.); acuity is measured by determining the most closely spaced lines (described as the highest frequency) for which the subject can discern the orientation

sinistro- prefix describing processes or structures occurring or appearing toward the left; in ophthalmic usage, part of the phrase oculus sinister, meaning the left eye; compare **dextro-**

sinus venosus sclerae see **Schlemm's canal**

Sjögren syndrome type of arthro-ophthalmopathy with ocular involvement including severe dry eye and fibrosis of the sclera

skew deviation see **deviation**

skiascopy see **retinoscopy**

slab-off lens bifocal lens in which a portion of the lower near-vision segment is ground away (thus the term slab-off) in such a way as to shift the optical center of that segment closer to the optical center of the upper distance vision part of the lens; this is important to balance the images provided by the two bifocal segments, which tend to be split because of the different refracting powers of the distance- and near-vision segments

slit lamp instrument that projects a beam of light onto the eye, usually as a narrow vertical beam (thus the term "slit") but with other beam shapes possible, allowing an examiner to view ocular structures through an attached low-power microscope; also called a biomicroscope

slit lamp biomicroscopy examination of a patient using the slit lamp

Sloan letters or **optotypes** block capital letters C, D, H, K, N, O, R, S, V and Z presented to a test subject at various sizes in a chart for testing distance vision and on cards for testing near vision

Snellen acuity measurement of visual acuity based upon standard sizes of letters visible to the "normal" eye at specified distances; the test type incorporated into Snellen's vision test target (introduced in chart form in the mid-1800s and in projector form in the 1920s) is the most commonly used "eye chart" in the U.S., and the standard testing distance of 20 feet gives us the familiar system of measuring distance visual acuity against a reference value of 20/20 (with 20/10 being extraordinarily sharp eyesight and larger denominators representing less accurate vision, down to a level of legal blindness generally defined at 20/200)

Snell's law optical formula defining the index of refraction of a substance as the sine of the angle of incidence divided by the sine of the angle of refraction

Soemmering's ring ring-shaped collection of crystalline lens material left after cataract extraction, which some times opacifies to form a Soemmering's ring cataract

soft contact lens see **contact lens**

soft exudates see **retinal exudates**

soft IOL see **intraocular lens**

spectacles eyeglasses; **aphakic s.** eyeglasses prescribed to correct vision after removal of a cataractous crystalline lens, usually requiring very thick lenses; **half-eye s.** spectacles incorporating semicircular lenses to allow the wearer to see the other half of the visual field unaided; **prismatic s.** see **prism**

spectrum see **electromagnetic spectrum**

specular microscopy technique for viewing the corneal endothelium, used to assess the health of the cornea, particularly around the time of ophthalmic surgery

speculum general term for an instrument that facilitates the observation of some part of the body; in ophthalmic usage, a lid speculum refers to a device placed during examination or surgery of the eye to hold the eyelids open

sphenoid bone one of the bones of the orbit

sphenoid fissure see **orbital fissure**

sphere 1. in optics, a lens whose surface is circular in cross-section in all directions; 2. in refraction, the component of refractive error that can be corrected with a spherical lens (myopia or hyperopia); compare **cylinder**

spherical aberration uneven refraction of light through a spherical lens in which rays of light traveling through the peripheral lens are not refracted to the same degree as rays traveling through more central portions

spherical equivalent 1. representation of the refractive power of a toric lens defined as the spherical power plus one half the cylinder power; 2. similar calculation performed on the components of a spectacle prescription to describe the overall refractive error of an eye

spherical lens lens in which all surfaces are circular in cross section

spherocylindrical see **toric lens**

sphincter general anatomic term for a circular muscle; in ophthalmic usage referring to the **pupillary sphincter**

sphincterotomy in ophthalmic usage, an incision into the pupillary sphincter, usually performed when a small pupil makes intraocular surgery more difficult

spindle cells see **Krukenberg's spindles**

spot retinoscope see **retinoscope**

squint see **strabismus**

squint angle see **angle of deviation**

staining see **corneal staining**

staphyloma thinning and protrusion of the sclera and/or cornea; **anterior s.** staphyloma around the cornea in the area of the ciliary body; **equatorial s.** staphyloma occurring midway between the anterior and posterior poles of the eye, usually where the vortex veins exit the globe; **posterior s.** staphyloma of the sclera in the posterior segment; **Scarpa's s.** posterior staphyloma occurring in extremely myopic eyes

static perimetry see **perimetry**

steep in ophthalmic usage, describing the surface curvature of a lens or ocular medium that imparts relatively large refractive power; compare **flat**

steep axis in a toric lens or spherocylindrical ocular medium, the axis opposite the cylinder

stenocoriasis constriction of the pupil

stenopeic general term applied to narrow, slit-like openings, as in a stenopeic lens

step see **nasal step**

stereopsis three-dimensional vision; see also **binocular vision** and **fusion**

stigmatic lens lens that brings light from a point source into a point of focus

stigmatoscopy technique for determining the refractive state of the eye by having the test subject view a pinpoint of light and report its appearance

strabismus misalignment of the visual axes of the eyes that impairs binocular vision; **absolute s.** strabismus present under all conditions and at all fixation distances; **accommodative s.** strabismus that occurs upon accommodation or attempted accommodation; **alternating s.** strabismus that affects each eye independently, so that either eye can maintain fixation at any time (also called **bilateral** or **binocular s.**); **anatomic s.** strabismus resulting from malformation of the structure of the eye, ocular muscles or orbit; **comitant** or **concomitant s.** strabismus in which the angle of deviation is the same for all directions of gaze and does not matter which eye is fixating; **constant s.** see **absolute s.; convergent s.** strabismus in which one or both eyes turn inward (also called **esotropia** or **internal strabismus**); **cyclic s.** strabismus that occurs and disappears at regular intervals of time; **divergent s.** strabismus in which one or both eyes turn outward (also called **exotropia** or **external strabismus**); **dynamic s.** muscular imbalance that tends to make the eye deviate but is usually overcome in normal binocular vision; **horizontal s.** strabismus in which the misalignment of the eyes is in a horizontal direction (compare **vertical s.**); **incomitant s.** strabismus in which the angle of deviation varies with the direction of gaze, fixating eye or fixation distance; **intermittent s.** strabismus that is not present at all times; **kinetic s.** strabismus resulting from spasm of the extraocular muscles; **latent s.** misalignment of the eye that occurs only when one eye is deprived of fusional stimulus (see **phoria**); **manifest s.** strabismus that is not latent; **mechanical s.** strabismus resulting from some anatomic pull upon or displacement of the eye or extraocular muscles; **microstrabismus** strabismus of such a small degree that it is only noted upon close examination; **muscular s.** strabismus resulting from some imbalance of the extraocular muscles; **monolateral** or **monocular s.** see **unilateral s.; noncomitant** or **nonconcomitant s.** see **incomitant s.; paralytic s.** strabismus resulting from paralysis of one or more extraocular muscles; **periodic** or **relative s.** strabismus that occurs only at certain directions of gaze or fixation distances; **spasmodic** or **spastic s.** strabismus resulting from spasm of one or more extraocular muscles; **suppressed s.** see **latent s.; unilateral s.** strabismus in which one eye deviates while the fellow eye achieves normal fixation; **vertical s.** strabismus in which the angle of deviation is in a vertical direction (compare **horizontal s.**); see also **angle of deviation, primary deviation** and **secondary deviation**

strabotomy surgical procedure to correct strabismus by cutting an extraocular muscle

streak retinoscopy see **retinoscopy**

striae general medical term for the appearance of lines or streaks in tissue; **corneal s.** lines in the cornea resulting from manipulation of ocular tissue, either temporary (as when instruments are being used during surgery) or permanent (as when a corneal incision is improperly closed); **retinal s.** lines visible in the retina following surgical or spontaneous reattachment of a detached retina

stroma general anatomic term for the structural element of a tissue or organ; **corneal s.** central layer of fibrous corneal tissue lying between Bowman's and Descemet's membranes; **iris s.** connective tissue to which the sphincter muscles, nerves and pigment of the iris adhere

Sturm's interval see **conoid of Sturm**

stye see **meibomian cyst**

subcapsular cataract see **cataract**

subchoroidal hemorrhage bleeding between the retina and choroid, leading to retinal detachment if left untreated (sometimes called suprachoroidal hemorrhage)

subconjunctival hemorrhage bleeding between the conjunctiva and sclera, dramatic in appearance (initially a blood-red patch on the surface of the eye) but usually posing no threat to eye or sight and resolves without treatment

subduction general term for downward motion; in ophthalmic usage, movement of the eye down toward the cheek

subjective refraction see **refraction**

subluxation general term for dislocation, as in a subluxated lens

substantia propria corneae and **sclerae** stroma of the cornea and sclera, respectively

sulcus general anatomic term describing a grooved or depressed area; see also **ciliary sulcus** and **scleral sulcus**

sulfur hexafluoride heavy gas used in surgery to repair retinal detachment

sunrise and **sunset syndromes** dislocation in which an intraocular lens is displaced upward or downward, respectively, in the pupil

supercilium proper term for the eyebrow and its surrounding area

superficial punctate keratitis see **keratitis**

superior oblique muscle extraocular muscle lying across the top of the eye responsible for depressing, abducting and intorting the eye

superior rectus muscle extraocular muscle lying across the top of the eye responsible for elevating, adducting and intorting the eye as well as raising the upper eyelid

suppression action of the brain to ignore the image from one eye during binocular vision as a result of anisometropia, deviation or other visual disturbance

suprachoroid the outer layer of the choroid and ciliary body consisting primarily of connective, avascular tissue

supraduction, supravergence, sursumduction and **sursumvergence** in ophthalmic usage, upward turning of one eye

supraorbital at the top of or above the bony eye socket

supraversion and **sursumversion** in ophthalmic usage, upward turning of both eyes

swinging flashlight test see **Marcus Gunn pupil**

symblepharon condition in which the conjunctiva of the eyelid adheres to the bulbar conjunctiva

sympathetic amaurosis see **amaurosis**

sympathetic ophthalmia rare condition in which trauma or intraocular foreign body leading to uveitis in one eye is followed by uveitis in the other, uninjured, eye; only removal of the injured eye will prevent loss of sight in both eyes

syncanthus adhesion of the tissues of the eye to the orbit in the area of the canthus

synchysis condition in which the vitreous humor loses its normal consistency and liquefies

synchysis scintillans formation of crystals within the vitreous humor

synechia general term for fibrous adhesion of organs or tissues; plural: synechiae; see also **peripheral anterior synechiae**

synechialysis surgical breaking of synechiae

syneresis in ophthalmic usage, degenerative shrinking of the vitreous body as a result of aging, often resulting in vitreous detachment

synoptophore table-top instrument that presents two separate fields of view to the eyes for testing binocular vision

Tt

tangential illumination in slit lamp biomicroscopy, method of viewing surfaces of ocular structures by shining light from the slit lamp light source at an angle across the surface of the structure

tarsal of or like the tarsus (eyelid)

tarsal angle see **canthus**

tarsal glands see **meibomian glands**

tarsal muscle one of the muscles in the eyelids, either upper (superior tarsal muscle, also called the **levator muscle**) or lower (inferior tarsal muscle)

tarsal plate see **tarsus**

tarsorrhaphy general term for surgical procedures in which the upper and lower eyelids are sutured together

tarsus "plate" of connective tissue that serves as the underlying structure of the eyelids, either upper (superior tarsus) or lower (inferior tarsus); plural: tarsi

tear break-up time see **break-up time**

tear duct, gland, etc. see **lacrimal apparatus**

tear film the natural fluid covering of the surface of the eye, composed primarily of three strata: an inner layer of mucin (produced in the conjunctival goblet cells), a middle watery layer (produced in the lacrimal glands, which also produce various important tear proteins like lactoferrin) and an outer layer of oily secretions (produced in the meibomian glands); contact lenses "ride" upon the tear film, which is constantly refreshed by the various glands mentioned above and continuously drains through the puncta and the nasolacrimal ducts into the nasal sinuses

telescope 1. general term for an optical device consisting of an objective (either a convex lens or concave mirror) and an ocular (a concave or convex lens) to enlarge and focus an image of a distant object; **Galilean t.** telescope in which the objective is a convex lens and the ocular is a concave lens, producing an erect image; 2. low-vision aid that employs telescopic optics to magnify a relatively narrow field of view

temple in opticianry, part of spectacle frame that rests against the head and usually extends over the ear

temporal general anatomic term for structure or process that appears or occurs on or toward the side of the head; see also **lateral;** compare **medial** and **nasal**

temporal canthus see **lateral canthus**

tenectomy surgical procedure in which a tendon is cut and removed (not to be confused with **tenonectomy**)

tenonectomy surgical removal of a portion of Tenon's capsule

tenonotomy surgical procedure in which an incision is made into Tenon's capsule

Tenon's capsule or **membrane** thin, outermost membrane of the eye, enclosing the entire globe except for the cornea

tenotomy surgical procedure in which a tendon is cut (not to be confused with **tenonotomy**)

thermokeratoplasty refractive surgical procedure to correct farsightedness in which heat is applied to the sclera at points around the cornea to shrink scleral tissue and thus steepen the cornea

thimerosal preservative used in some topical ophthalmic medications and contact lens care solutions

tonic pupil see **pupil**

tonography measurement taken by a tonometer

tonometer instrument that measures intraocular pressure; **air-puff t.** see **pneumotonometer**; **applanation t.** tonometer that measures intraocular pressure by quantifying the resistance of the eye to flattening, typically incorporating concentric ring markings that show the amount of ocular surface area that is flattened, with greater flattening indicating lower intraocular pressure (also called applanometer); **Goldmann t.** classic applanation tonometer design incorporated into slit lamps; **indentation t.** tonometer that measures intraocular pressure by quantifying the degree to which the eye can be indented, for example, the **Schiotz tonometer; noncontact t.** see **pneumotonometer; pneumotonometer** type of noncontact tonometer that uses a puff of air to measure intraocular pressure

tonometry the act of measuring intraocular pressure using a tonometer; **digital t.** method of measuring approximate intraocular pressure by pressing against the eye with a finger

Tono-Pen brand name of tonometer that gives an electronic readout of intraocular pressure when a probe is placed against the globe

topography see **corneal topography**

toric lens spectacle or contact lens having spherical and cylindrical components of curvature, prescribed to correct vision in an eye with astigmatism that is also myopic or hyperopic; see also **aspheric, bifocal lens** and **multifocal lens**

trabecular meshwork in ophthalmic usage, the structure at the junction of the ciliary body and sclera through which aqueous humor drains from the anterior chamber of the eye

trabeculectomy general term for a surgical procedure in which tissue is removed from the trabecular meshwork, most often to treat glaucoma by allowing aqueous humor to drain more easily from the eye

trabeculoplasty general term for surgical procedures, most commonly describing laser surgical procedures such as **argon laser trabeculoplasty,** that attempt to modify the structure of the trabecular meshwork and increase the outflow of aqueous humor in eyes with glaucoma

trabeculotomy general term for a surgical procedure involving an incision into the trabecular meshwork

trachoma inflammation of the cornea and conjunctiva caused by infection with chlamydia organisms, leading to blindness if not treated

traction retinal detachment see **retinal detachment**

transillumination in slit lamp biomicroscopy, evaluation of an ocular structure (often the lens and iris) by noting how light passes through it

traumatic cataract see **cataract**

trephine surgical instrument consisting of an open cylinder with a sharp end for cutting a circular incision, typically used in ophthalmic surgery to make an incision around the edge of the cornea so it can be removed; see also **penetrating keratoplasty**

trial frame specially designed spectacle frame in which various trial lenses can be placed to determine the power of lens needed to correct visual defect

trial lens 1. spectacle lenses used in a trial frame; 2. contact lenses used to check the fit before prescribing final lenses

trichiasis condition in which the lashes are turned inward toward the globe (as in entropion) and irritate ocular surface tissues

trifocal lens spectacle lens with three different segments that focus at near, medium and far distances; also see bifocal lens

trochlea ring of cartilaginous tissue attached to the frontal bone, through which passes the tendon of the superior oblique muscle

tropia misalignment of the eyes in which they fail to fixate on the same object; see also **strabismus**

troposcope table-top instrument that presents two separate fields of view to the eyes for testing binocular vision

truncation method of stabilizing toric contact lenses by "cutting off" one or two edges of the lens so that it is no longer circular, thereby creating a linear edge that rests against the lid margin and possibly provides greater adherence to the eye; truncation is employed to help prevent rotation and maintain the orientation of toric contact lenses to correct astigmatism in the proper axis; compare **dynamic stabilization, posterior toric** and **prism ballast**

tunnel vision visual field defect in which only a small central portion of the visual field remains functional

typoscope low-vision aid consisting of a rectangle of dark, nonreflective material with a narrow horizontal slit through which type can be read, thereby minimizing glare from the page and isolating the words being read

Uu

UGH syndrome inflammatory condition of internal ocular structures occurring as a complication of intraocular lens implantation, consisting of uveitis, glaucoma and hyphema

ultraviolet portion of the electromagnetic spectrum with short wavelengths, not visible to the human eye; abbreviated UV, ultraviolet radiation causes sunburn and tanning, and has been implicated in certain ocular conditions, most notably cataract formation

ultraviolet A and B the two bands of ultraviolet radiation

ultraviolet blocker substance incorporated into spectacle, contact and intraocular lenses to eliminate the ultraviolet component of sunlight reaching the eye

uncorrected visual acuity visual acuity measured without corrective lenses in place (abbreviation: VA_{sc}); compare **best corrected visual acuity**

undercorrection state in which the power of corrective lenses or the effect of refractive surgery is insufficient to achieve the desired visual acuity; compare **overcorrection**

unilateral general anatomic term describing a structure or process appearing or occurring on only one side; in ophthalmic usage, referring to a single eye; see also **monocular;** compare **binocular**

uniocular see **monocular**

uvea the tissues of the eye that are heavily pigmented and consist primarily of blood vessels; the choroid, ciliary body and iris considered as a whole system

uveitis inflammation of all or part of the uvea; **anterior u.** uveitis involving only the iris and ciliary body; **phacolytic u.** uveitis resulting from degeneration and leakage of lens tissue; **posterior u.** uveitis involving only the choroid

Vv

Van Lint block injection of anesthetic agents to achieve akinesia (prevention of movement) of the eyelids

vault see definition 1 under **apical clearance**

vergence 1. in optics, the gathering together or spreading apart of parallel light rays, either naturally or as a result of passing through a lens; 2. in ophthalmic usage, motion of the eyes toward or away from one another; see also **convergence** and **divergence**

vernal conjunctivitis see **conjunctivitis**

version coordinated movement of both eyes in the same direction

vertex distance distance along the line of sight from the cornea to the back surface of a spectacle lens

vertex power focusing power of a spectacle lens measured from either of its surfaces; **back v.p.** portion of the total refractive power imparted by the posterior surface of a lens; **front v.p.** portion of the total refractive power imparted by the anterior surface of a lens

videokeratography see **corneal topography**

viscodissection surgical technique in which a viscoelastic substance is injected between tissues (commonly the tissues surrounding the lens nucleus) in order to separate them and facilitate subsequent manipulation

viscoelastic material any one of a number of thick gels manufactured for use in ophthalmic surgery, injected into the eye to help maintain the shape of ocular structures and as a lubricant/coating to minimize trauma from surgical instruments and implants; currently used viscoelastic materials include chondroitin sulfate, hyaluronic acid and methylcellulose, used individually or in combination and marketed under several brand names

vision action of the eyes, nervous system and brain in capturing reflected light from the environment and converting it to perceived images; see also **binocular v., distance v., low v., night v.,** etc.

vision training any of several systems employing ocular exercises to enhance development or correct deficiencies of stereopsis, hand-eye coordination, etc.

visual acuity clarity of vision; specifically, the ability to distinguish fine details, often expressed as a score on Snellen, Jaeger, or other vision test charts; **best corrected v.a.** highest level of visual acuity that can be attained with corrective lenses in place (abbreviation: BCVA); **corrected v.a.** visual acuity measured with corrective lenses in place (abbreviation: VA_{cc}); **uncorrected v.a.** visual acuity measured without corrective lenses in place (abbreviation: UCVA or VA_{sc})

visual axis imaginary line traced from the fovea to the object of fixation, commonly called the line of sight

visual evoked potential or **visual evoked response** fluctuation in brain activity that results from a visual stimulus, measurable on electroencephalography

visual field 1. area around the fixation point of each eye in which objects can be seen, generally circular in shape; 2. in clinical usage, graphs representing the result of perimetry and other such tests are often simply referred to as visual fields; visual field testing is often conducted to determine areas of the retina that have been damaged by glaucoma or retinal detachment, as well as to determine any portions of the optic nerve tract that might be compromised by trauma or disease; see also **hemianopia, perimetry, quadrantanopia** and **scotoma**

visual field defect area of diminished or absent vision within the visual field

vitrectomy surgical procedure involving partial or total removal of vitreous humor and any membranes, blood or other tissue in the posterior chamber; **anterior v.** vitrectomy carried out as part of anterior segment surgery without entering the posterior chamber, usually considered to be a complication; **automated v.** vitrectomy performed using a cutting probe with irrigation and aspiration capabilities; **complete v.** removal of all vitreous from the posterior chamber; **manual v.**

vitrectomy performed using scissors rather than a vitrector; **open-sky v.** vitrectomy performed by opening the cornea and removing the lens; **pars plana v.** vitrectomy performed by making small incisions and inserting instruments through the pars plana; **partial v.** removal of only part of the vitreous humor from the posterior chamber; **scissors v.** see **manual v.**; **total v.** see **complete v.**

vitrector surgical instrument designed for performing vitrectomy, incorporating a cutting probe with irrigation and aspiration capabilities

vitreous body or **humor** clear, fibrous, gel-like material filling the posterior chamber of the eye, located behind the iris and lens capsule and comprising about two-thirds of the total volume of the eye, typically referred to simply as the vitreous; compare **aqueous humor**

vitreous detachment separation of all or part of the vitreous humor from its natural attachments to the retina

vitreous face see **hyaloid membrane**

vitreous floaters see **floaters**

vitreous membrane see **hyaloid membrane**

vitreous strands appearance of vitreous humor in the anterior chamber as strands of viscous, transparent tissue still attached to the hyaloid membrane

vitreous tap diagnostic procedure in which a small amount of vitreous humor is removed for testing, usually to perform a culture to confirm the existence and cause of infection

von Graefe's sign delay in or absence of downward motion of upper eyelid when the eye looks downward, a result of Graves' disease (which involves serious dysfunction of the thyroid gland)

vortex veins veins formed by the joining of veins draining blood from the iris, ciliary body and choroid exiting the eye through the sclera just posterior to the equator of the globe

Ww

wall-eye see **exotropia**

Weck-cel sponge brand name of a widely used surgical instrument consisting of a wedge of cellulose sponge mounted on a short handle; some procedures, most notably Weck-cel vitrectomy, in which the sponge plays a major role are identified using the term

wet macular degeneration see **macular degeneration**

wetting angle angle made by the surface of a drop of water and the surface of the material on which the drop lies; the larger the contact angle (up to a theoretical maximum of 90°), the less hydrophilic or "wettable" is the material; usually applied in ophthalmic usage as a description of contact lens materials

white-to-white measurement size of the cornea measured as the distance from a point just on the edge of the white tissue of the sclera to a similar point diametrically opposite

with-the-rule astigmatism see **astigmatism**

word blindness see **alexia**

Worth four-dot test test of binocular vision in which four dots, colored white, red and green, are presented to a test subject who views them through two filters, one red and the other green, placed before the eyes

Xx

xenon photocoagulator device that produces intensely bright light, with ophthalmic applications similar to lasers

xenophthalmia general term for unhealthy condition of an eye attributable to the presence of a foreign body

xerophthalmia dry eye condition resulting from vitamin A deficiency

Yy

YAG laser see **Nd:YAG laser** under **laser**

yoke muscles extraocular muscles of each eye that are neurologically paired so that they coordinate motion of both eyes in the same direction; see also **Hering's law of simultaneous innervation**

Y-sutures of crystalline lens tissue structure of the crystalline lens in which the ends of lens fibers join to form a Y shape

Zz

zeisian glands oil-producing glands within the eyelids at the base of the eyelashes

Zeiss lens see **goniolens**

zonules fibers that attach the edge of the lens capsule to the ciliary body

zonulolysis or **zonulysis** breakage of the zonules, occurring either naturally, from trauma or through intentional or unintentional surgical manipulation

zygomatic bone one of the bones of the orbit

Abbreviations Commonly Used in Ophthalmic Practice

AA	accommodation amplitude
AACAHPO	American Association of Certified Allied Health Personnel in Ophthalmology
AAO	American Academy of Ophthalmology or American Academy of Optometry
ABES	American Board of Eye Surgeons
ABO	American Board of Ophthalmology or American Board of Opticianry
a.c.	before meals (often in prescriptions)
AC	anterior chamber
AC/A ratio	accommodative convergence/accommodation ratio
ACES	American College of Eye Surgeons
ACG	angle-closure glaucoma; see glaucoma
AC IOL	anterior chamber intraocular lens (equivalent to ACL); see intraocular lens
ACL	anterior chamber lens (equivalent to AC IOL); see intraocular lens
ACS	American College of Surgeons or Automated Corneal Shaper microkeratome (trademark)
AK	astigmatic keratotomy; see keratotomy

ALK	automated lamellar keratoplasty; see keratoplasty
ALT	argon laser trabeculoplasty; see trabeculoplasty
AMA	American Medical Association
AMD	age-related macular degeneration (also ARMD); see macular degeneration
AMO	Allergan Medical Optics (company name)
ANSI	American National Standards Institute
AOA	American Optometric Association
ARC	anomalous (or abnormal) retinal correspondence
ARMD	age-related macular degeneration (also AMD); see macular degeneration
asb	apostilb
ASCRS	American Society of Cataract and Refractive Surgery
ASICO	American Surgical Instrument Company (company name)
ATR	against-the-rule; see astigmatism
AUPO	Association of University Professors in Ophthalmology
BAK	benzalkonium chloride
BAT	Brightness Acuity Tester (trademark)
BCVA	best corrected visual acuity
b.i.d.	twice per day (often in prescriptions)

BIOM	Binocular Indirect Ophthalmic Microscope (trademark)
BO	base-out; see prism
BRA	branch retinal artery
BRAO	branch retinal artery occlusion
BRV	branch retinal vein
BRVO	branch retinal vein occlusion
BSS	Balanced Salt Solution (trademark, but often used as generic)
BUVA	best uncorrected visual acuity
BUT	break-up time (of tear film)
BVD	back vertex power
c or cum	with (often in prescriptions)
CAI	carbonic anhydrase inhibitor
cd	candela
CF	count-finger vision (visual acuity)
C_3F_8	perfluoropropane; see perfluorocarbon
CL	contact lens
CLAO	Contact Lens Association of Ophthalmologists
cm	centimeter
CME	cystoid macular edema
CMV	cytomegalovirus; see retinitis
CNV	choroidal neovascularization
CO	Certified Orthoptist
COA	Certified Ophthalmic Assistant
COAG	chronic open-angle glaucoma; see glaucoma
coll or collyr	eyewash (often in prescriptions)

COMT	Certified Ophthalmic Medical Technologist
COT	Certified Ophthalmic Technician
CRA	central retinal artery
CRAO	central retinal artery occlusion
CRNO	Certified Registered Nurse in Ophthalmology
CRV	central retinal vein
CRVO	central retinal vein occlusion
cyl	cylinder
d	day (often in prescriptions)
D	diopter
DCR	dacryocystorhinostomy
DR	diabetic retinopathy
DVD	dissociated vertical deviation; see deviation
ECCE	extracapsular cataract extraction
EDTA	ethylenediamine tetra-acetic acid
EOG	electro-oculography
EOM	extraocular muscle(s)
ERG	electroretinography
ET	esotropia
FAAO	Fellow of the American Academy of Ophthalmology or Fellow of the American Academy of Optometry
FACS	Fellow of the American College of Surgeons
FRCP	Fellow of the Royal College of Physicians (of England); may be followed by (A) for Australia or (C) for Canada

FRCS	Fellow of the Royal College of Surgeons (of England); may be followed by (A) for Australia or (C) for Canada
GPC	giant papillary conjunctivitis; see conjunctivitis
gt	drop (often in prescriptions)
gtt	drops (often in prescriptions)
h	hour (often in prescriptions)
HEMA	hydroxyethylmethacrylate, see hydrogel
HM	hand-motion vision (visual acuity)
HOTV	HOTV test
h.s.	at bedtime (often in prescriptions)
HSK	herpes simplex keratitis; see herpes keratitis under keratitis
IA, I&A or I/A	irrigation and aspiration
ICCE	intracapsular cataract extraction
ICE	iridocorneal endothelial syndrome
ICL	Implantable Contact Lens (trademark)
ICR	intrastromal corneal ring (trade name)
Ig	immunoglobulin
ILM	internal limiting membrane of the retina
IO	inferior oblique muscle
IOFB	intraocular foreign body, see foreign body
IOL	intraocular lens

ION	ischemic optic neuropathy
IOP	intraocular pressure
IR	inferior rectus muscle
ISRS	International Society of Refractive Surgery
J	Jaeger (visual) acuity
JCAHPO	Joint Commission on Allied Health Personnel in Ophthalmology
K	keratometry
KCS	keratoconjunctivitis sicca
KP	keratic precipitates
KPE	Kelman phacoemulsification
LASIK	laser in situ keratomileusis
LE	left eye
LEC	lens epithelial cell(s)
LIO	laser indirect ophthalmoscope; see indirect ophthalmoscopy
LP	light perception vision (visual acuity)
LR	lateral rectus muscle
LTK	laser thermokeratoplasty
LVS	Low Vision Specialist
LXT	left exotropia
m	meter
MR	medial rectus muscle
MTF	modulation transfer function
N or n	refractive index
NCLE	National Contact Lens Examiners
Nd:YAG	neodymium:yttrium-aluminum-garnet laser
NEI	National Eye Institute
NFL	nerve fiber layer (of retina)

NIH	National Institutes of Health
NLP	no light perception vision
nm	nanometer
NPA	near point of accommodation
NPC	near point of convergence
n.p.o.	nothing by mouth (often in prescriptions)
NRC	normal retinal correspondence
NSPB	National Society for the Prevention of Blindness
NVG	neovascular glaucoma
OA	Ophthalmic Assistant or Optometric Assistant
OAG	open-angle glaucoma
OCT	Optical Coherence Tomographer (trademark)
OD	oculus dexter (right eye)
OEP	Optometric Extension Program
OHT	ocular hypertension
OOSS	Outpatient Ophthalmic Surgery Society
OPMI	microscope (trademark)
OS	oculus sinister (left eye)
OT	Ophthalmic Technician or Optometric Technician
OU	oculi uterque (each eye or both eyes)
OZ	optical zone
PAM	Potential Acuity Meter (trademark)
PARK	photorefractive astigmatic keratectomy

PAS	peripheral anterior synechiae
PBK	pseudophakic bullous keratopathy
p.c.	after meals (often in prescriptions)
PC	posterior chamber
PC IOL	posterior chamber intraocular lens (equivalent to PCL); see intraocular lens
PCL	posterior chamber lens (equivalent to PC IOL); see intraocular lens
PCO	posterior capsule opacification; see capsule
PD	pupillary distance or prism diopter
PI	peripheral iridotomy or peripheral iridectomy
PKP	penetrating keratoplasty; see keratoplasty
PMMA	polymethylmethacrylate
p.o.	by mouth (often in prescriptions)
POAG	primary open-angle glaucoma
PRK	photorefractive keratectomy
p.r.n.	as needed (often in prescriptions)
PRP	panretinal photocoagulation
PSC	posterior subcapsular cataract
PTK	phototherapeutic keratectomy
PVD	posterior vitreous detachment
PVR	proliferative vitreoretinopathy
q.2h.	every 2 hours (often in prescriptions)
q.d.	every day (often in prescriptions)
q.h.	every hour (often in prescriptions)
q.i.d.	four times per day (often in prescriptions)

q.s.	as much as needed (often in prescriptions)
RD	retinal detachment
RE	right eye
RGP	rigid gas-permeable lens; see contact lens
RHT	right hypertropia
RK	radial keratotomy
ROP	retinopathy of prematurity
RP	retinitis pigmentosa
RPE	retinal pigment epithelium
s or sine	without (often in prescriptions)
SCL	soft contact lens; see contact lens
SE	spherical equivalent
SF_6	sulfur hexafluoride
sig.	instructions (often in prescriptions)
SO	superior oblique muscle
sol.	solution (often in prescriptions)
SPK	superficial punctate keratitis
SR	superior rectus muscle
susp.	suspension (often in prescriptions)
T	tropia
tab.	tablet (often in prescriptions)
t.i.d.	three times per day (often in prescriptions)
TK	thermokeratoplasty
UGH	uveitis-glaucoma-hyphema (syndrome)
ung.	ointment (often in prescriptions)
ut dict	as directed (often in prescriptions)

UV	ultraviolet
UVA	ultraviolet band A
UVB	ultraviolet band B
VA	visual acuity
VA_{cc}	corrected visual acuity
VA_{sc}	uncorrected visual acuity
VEP	visual evoked potential
VER	visual evoked response
VF	visual field
W4D	Worth four-dot test
WTR	with-the-rule; see astigmatism
XT	exotropia
YAG	see Nd:YAG laser under laser